EMBRYO CLEAVAGE

Edited by **Bin Wu**

Embryo Cleavage
http://dx.doi.org/10.5772/65555
Edited by Bin Wu

Contributors

Meng Ju Lee, Juan Carlos Fierro-González, Anna Leida, Aisha Khan, Gabor Laszlo Kovacs, Gergely Montsko, Zita Zrinyi, Akos Varnagy, Jozsef Bodis, Pinar Tulay, Nasim Tabibnejad, Bin Wu

Published by InTech
Janeza Trdine 9, 51000 Rijeka, Croatia

Publishing Process Manager Romina Skomersic
Technical Editor SPi Global
Cover InTech Design team

First published September, 2017
Printed in Croatia
Legal deposit, Croatia: National and University Library in Zagreb

Additional hard copies can be obtained from orders@intechopen.com

Embryo Cleavage, Edited by Bin Wu
p. cm.
Print ISBN 978-953-51-3511-1
Online ISBN 978-953-51-3512-8

For EU product safety concerns:
IN TECH d.o.o., Prolaz Marije Krucifikse Kozulić 3, 51000 Rijeka, Croatia,
info@intechopen.com or visit our website at intechopen.com.

Meet the editor

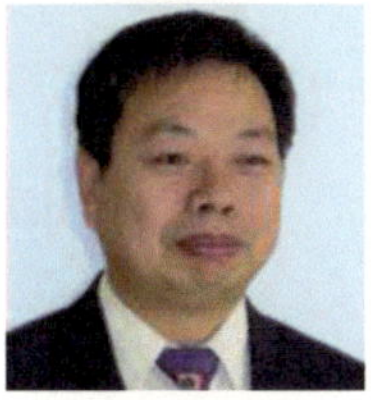

Bin Wu, PhD, HCLD, is currently a scientific laboratory director at Arizona Center for Reproductive Endocrinology and Infertility, USA. He received his training in genetics and reproductive biology at the Northwest Agricultural University in China and Cornell University, New York, and his postdoctoral training at the University of Guelph, Canada. He was promoted as a professor at the Northwest Agricultural University. As an embryologist, he later joined the Center for Human Reproduction in Chicago. Dr. Wu has membership for many professional associations, such as American Society for Reproductive Medicine, International Embryo Transfer Society, Society for the Study of Reproduction, American Association of Bioanalysts, and European Society of Human Reproduction and Embryology. Also, he has obtained some significant research awards from these professional associations. American College of Embryology recognizes Dr. Wu's excellence in the practice of Reproductive Embryology of the following practitioner in July 2014. He has edited books entitled Advances in Embryo Transfer (English and Chinese edition) and New Discoveries in Embryology in InTech, which have been downloaded more than 10,000 times.

Contents

Preface

Embryo cleavage is the division of cells in the early embryo. This division from one-celled zygote into two cells, four cells, eight cells, and sixteen cells, morula stage, and the final forming blastocyst stage until implanting in the uterus is called embryo cleavage. These stage embryos still do not implant in the uterus, and also they are called as preimplantation embryos. Preimplantation embryo development experiences a series of critical events and remarkable epigenetic modifications, and reprogramming of gene expression occurs to activate the embryonic genome. The development of current assisted reproductive technology (ART) has created some new observations and novel discoveries in cleavage embryos. For example, in order to observe embryo morphology and assess embryo quality, time-lapse imaging and light-sheet microscopy have made it possible to visualize early mammalian development in greater detail and over longer time periods than ever before. Thus, this book will collect some new technologies and methods on the study of cleavage embryos to select high-quality embryos for transfer and improve embryo implantation and pregnancy.

Since the birth of the first in vitro fertilization (IVF or test-tube) baby, ART has been widely used in human infertility treatment and animal population reproduction and expansion. However, the success of assisted reproductive technology mainly depends on the production of viable embryos with high implantation potential. More importantly, choosing the best embryo for transfer has become the major challenge in IVF. In the early embryo culture, the embryo quality assessment was mainly based on the morphological criteria of transfer embryo. Thus, performing serial observation of embryo morphology is a common technique for embryologist to evaluate embryos and has been considered as key predictor of implantation and pregnancy. For a long term, embryologists perform embryo quality and morphology assessment by taking embryos out of incubator and placing under a microscope. However, although this is easily practiced, it frequently takes embryos out of incubator due to concerns for safety and stability of culture conditions. Also, some key points of embryonic development may be missed for observation. Recently, various time lapse microscopy incubators have started to be used in human IVF clinic to monitor all steps of embryo growth and development. Time-lapse imaging is another noninvasive, emerging technology that allows 24-hour monitoring of embryo development, offering the possibility of increased quantity and quality of morphological information without disturbing the culture condition. This technique has been able to improve transferred embryo implantation and pregnancy. Thus, in the second part of this book, some morphokinetic markers can be revealed in time-lapse system. The first is the time outline of embryo cleavage, and embryologists may clearly know what situation embryo should be at various time points. Thus, an optimal quality embryo or high potential implantation embryo may be selected for transfer to obtain a higher pregnancy rate. Secondly, some specific events (such as a four-dimensional video sequencing of embryos) of cleavage embryos may be observed by morphokinetic markers and spatiotemporal analysis and innovated computer hardware and software analysis to determine embryo developmental speed, sex, etc. Simultaneous monitoring of molecular processes enables the study of connections between genetic expression and cell physiology and development.

Cleavage embryos experience a series of gene expression. In the early stages, maternal mRNAs direct embryonic development. New study showed that differential demethylation process results in differential parental gene expression in the early developing embryos that may have an impact on the correct development. Thus, Part III listed a review paper that showed different factors affecting gene expression during early embryo development, which included epigenetic factors, focusing on methylation profiles. The effects of noncoding RNAs on gene expression were thoroughly evaluated. Based on the products of gene expression, an available metabolic and proteomic approach as the noninvasive molecular assessment of embryo viability has been described. A new discovery, the alpha-1 chain of the human haptoglobin molecule, may be used as a quantitative biomarker of embryo viability. If this molecular composition of cultivation media can be used as an additional noninvasive procedure to choose an embryo for selective transfer, it will be very useful to improve human IVF pregnancy outcome.

Embryonic quality, cleavage speed, and gene expression have a close relationship with in vitro culture environment, including culture media, incubator type, and gas concentration. Thus, an optimum for embryo in vitro culture plays important roles in improving embryo quality and pregnancy rate. In the last part of this book, an interesting research report has been listed, which showed the favorable response of individual patient's embryos to media and incubators. Some patents' embryos grow very well in one kind of medium, but it does not grow well in the other medium. Thus, in human IVF clinic practice, using two media and two incubators for embryo culture could significantly improve IVF/ICSI embryo quality and increase pregnant rates.

I thank all authors who devoted their time and expertise to prepare these outstanding chapters included in this book.

Bin Wu, PhD, HCLD (ABB)
Arizona Center for Reproductive Endocrinology and Infertility
Tucson, Arizona
USA

Section 1

Introductory

Chapter 1

Introductory Chapter: New Technologies for the Study of Embryo Cleavage

Bin Wu

Additional information is available at the end of the chapter

http://dx.doi.org/10.5772/intechopen.69382

1. Introduction

After fertilization by sperm into oocyte combination, mammal embryogenesis is the process of cell division and cellular differentiation of the embryo that occurs during the early stages of development. In embryology, cleavage is the division of cells in the early embryo. This division from a one-celled zygote into 2, 4, 8, and 16 cells; morula stage; and finally into blastocyst stage until implantation in the uterus is called embryo cleavage. The zygotes of many species undergo rapid cell cycles with no significant growth, producing a cluster of cells the same size as the original zygote. The different cells derived from the cleavage are called blastomeres and form a compact mass called the morula. Cleavage ends with the formation of the blastula known as the blastocyst stage embryo that is yet to implant in the uterus and hence is also called preimplantation embryo.

In the last three decades, the development of assisted reproductive technology (ART) has created some new observations and novel discoveries in preimplantation embryos, especially during embryo cleavage. Preimplantation embryo development experiences a series of critical events and remarkable epigenetic modifications, and reprogramming of gene expression occurs to activate the embryonic genome. The alteration of these events often results in changes of embryo quality and morphology. At the cleavage stage, although morphological scores assigned using traditional criteria have little relationship with chromosome abnormalities [1], morphological evaluation is a major tool to assess embryo quality. Thus, many new observations and technologies have been developed. For example, in order to observe embryo morphology and to assess embryo quality, time-lapse imaging, and light-sheet microscopy have made it possible to visualize early mammalian development in greater detail and over longer time periods than ever before [2–4]. This book collects some new technologies and methods on the study of cleavage embryos to select high-quality embryos for transfer and to improve embryo implantation and pregnancy.

2. Observation of fertilized embryos to cleavage embryos

Since the first rabbit embryo culture was described in 1912 [5] and mouse zygote could be cultured in vitro to form blastocyst stage embryos [6, 7], embryo quality has become an important factor for pregnancy after the transfer of in vitro embryo into the uterus because embryo quality has a close correlation with transferred embryo implantation in uterus. Since the birth of the first "test-tube" baby, Louise Brown in July 1978, for which the 2010 Nobel Prize for Physiology or Medicine was awarded to Robert Edwards for developing in vitro fertilization (IVF) and embryo transfer (ET) to treat infertility in women with non-patent oviducts, in vitro embryo production (IVP) has been widely used in human infertility treatment and animal population reproduction and expansion. However, the success of assisted reproductive technology mainly depends on the production of viable embryos with high implantation potential. More importantly, choosing the best embryo for transfer has become the major challenge in IVF. In the early embryo culture, the embryo quality assessment was mainly based on the morphological criteria of the transferred embryo. Thus, performing a serial observation of embryo morphology is a common technique for embryologists to evaluate embryos and has been considered as a key predictor of implantation and pregnancy [8–10]. For a long term, embryologists performed embryo quality and morphology assessments by taking the embryos out of the incubator and placing under a microscope. Besides morphology observation, the researchers are interested in a series of studies on cell nuclear change, gene activation and expression, cytoplasmic protein expression, blastomere differentiation, and so on. However, these studies often result in the death of embryos. For example, in our early study which observed microspindle change after the sperm entry into the egg or the activation of oocyte, the fertilized zygotes or activated eggs needed to be fixed on the slide and stained with immunocytochemical fluorescein and laser confocal microscopy [11]. Our research clearly showed the alteration of microtubule and chromatin after bovine oocyte activation and introcytoplasmic sperm injection (ICSI; **Figure 1**). The sperm into oocyte or calcium ionophore and ethanol may activate oocyte and cause extrusion of the second polar body. In order to observe the time of the second polar body, we stained various stages of oocytes after activation. The result showed that after 5-hour postactivation, the second polar body may be completely extruded (**Figure 2**).

The study of gene expression often requires to isolate mRNA or protein from embryos [12–14]; hence, embryos needed to be lysed and no embryo would survive. In order to study the cell differentiation on moral and blastocyst stage embryos, a double staining with fluorescein microscopy method has been used to distinguish inner cell mass (ICM) from trophoectoderm (TE). The numbers of two different cells may be counted based on different colors (ICM as blue and TE as pink, **Figure 3**).

These research methods finally damage all embryos, and it is impossible to apply these methods to clinical practice. Thus, current embryo quality assessment is based primarily on the morphological criteria of transferred embryos, which includes three major parameters such as blastomere regularity, fragmentation, and cytoplasmic granularity [15]. Also, embryo cell numbers on different culture day and multinuclearity can be considered to evaluate embryo quality [16, 17]. Several reports have documented the association between the morphological

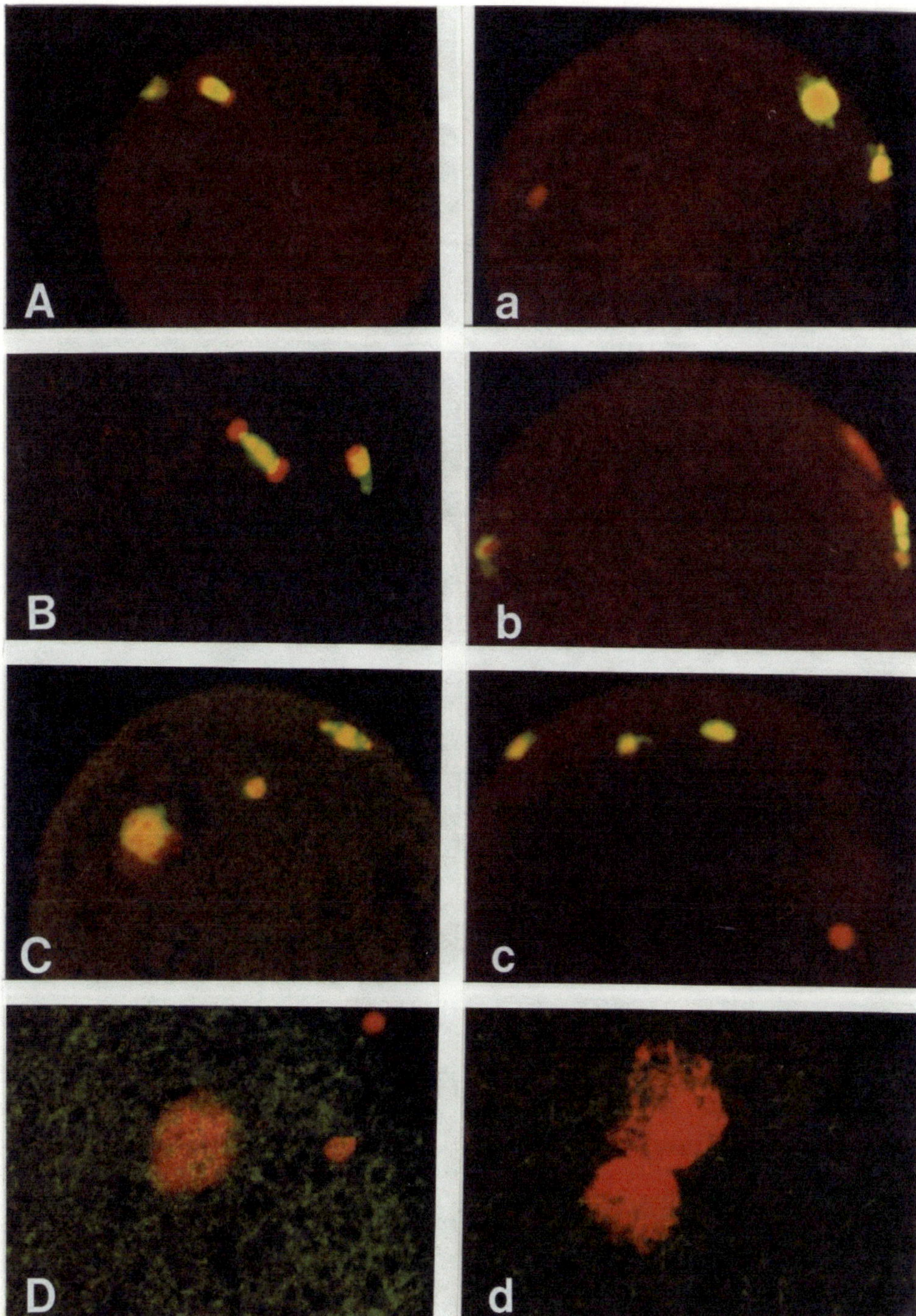

Figure 1. Laser-scanning confocal microscopy of spindle and chromatin changes at the various time post-activation and intracytoplasmic sperm injection (ICSI) in bovine. Capital letters (Left) indicate the change post-activation and small letters (Right) indicate after ICSI. A/a showed at 0.5 h, B/b is 2 h, C/c is 3 h, and D/d is 7 h post-activation or ICSI. Prenucleus in activated egg and prenuclei in ICSI egg have appeared with red color.

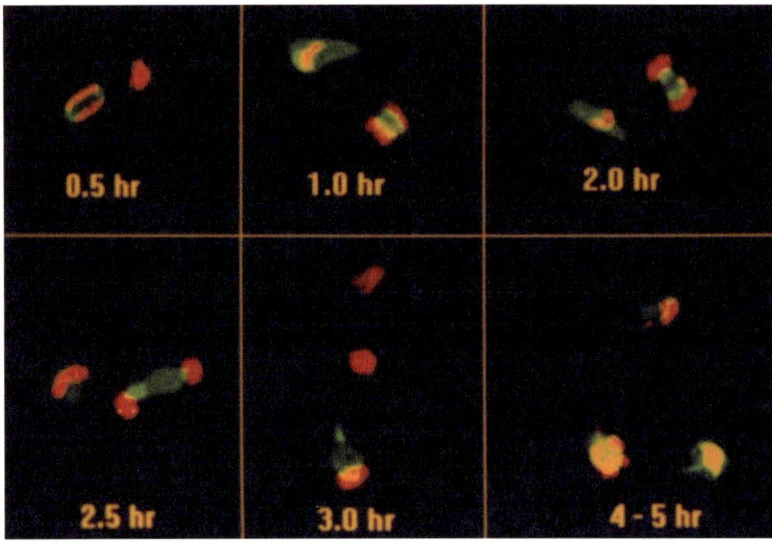

Figure 2. Laser-scanning confocal microscopy of spindle and chromatin changes at the various times post activation in bovine. At 0.5 h after activation, the chromosomes of spindle start to divide, and the completion of spindle division needs about 3 hours and the second polar body may be extruded at about 5 hours. The red and green together indicate the spindle, and the red point indicates the first polar body.

characteristics of cleavage stage embryos with pregnancy success. Thus, this is currently the basic method for embryo quality assessment in human IVF and animal in vitro embryo production. However, although this is easily practiced, it frequently takes embryos out of the incubator which leads to concerns for the safety and stability of culture conditions [18]. Also, some key points of embryonic development may be missed during observation. Evaluation of cleavage embryos during culture and before embryo transfer is an important clinical practice. Currently, the major assessment of in vitro fertilized embryos is visual observation using microscopy. In recent years, various time-lapse microscopy incubators are being used in human IVF clinic to monitor all the steps of embryo growth and development. Although preimplantation embryo diagnosis and screen (PGD/PGS) technologies have been applied in human embryo selection practice to improve pregnancy rate, these techniques are invasive for embryos. Finding another noninvasive method to select a good embryo will be very useful in human ART practice. Sallam et al. [19] reviewed noninvasive methods for embryo selection and evaluated these methods in the light of the best currently available evidence to find out whether any of them is ripe for replacing or supplementing the time-honored method of morphological assessment. Thus, we need more powerful tools to estimate the morphokinetic markers of embryos.

2.1. Embryo cleavage morphokinetics based on time-lapse imaging

For decades, researchers have attempted to follow the development of multicellular organisms from fertilized eggs into adults. While scientists had explored individual steps of this process, no method existed to enable them to model the whole process of development live. Currently, advances in light-sheet microscopy reported in two *Nature Methods* papers have

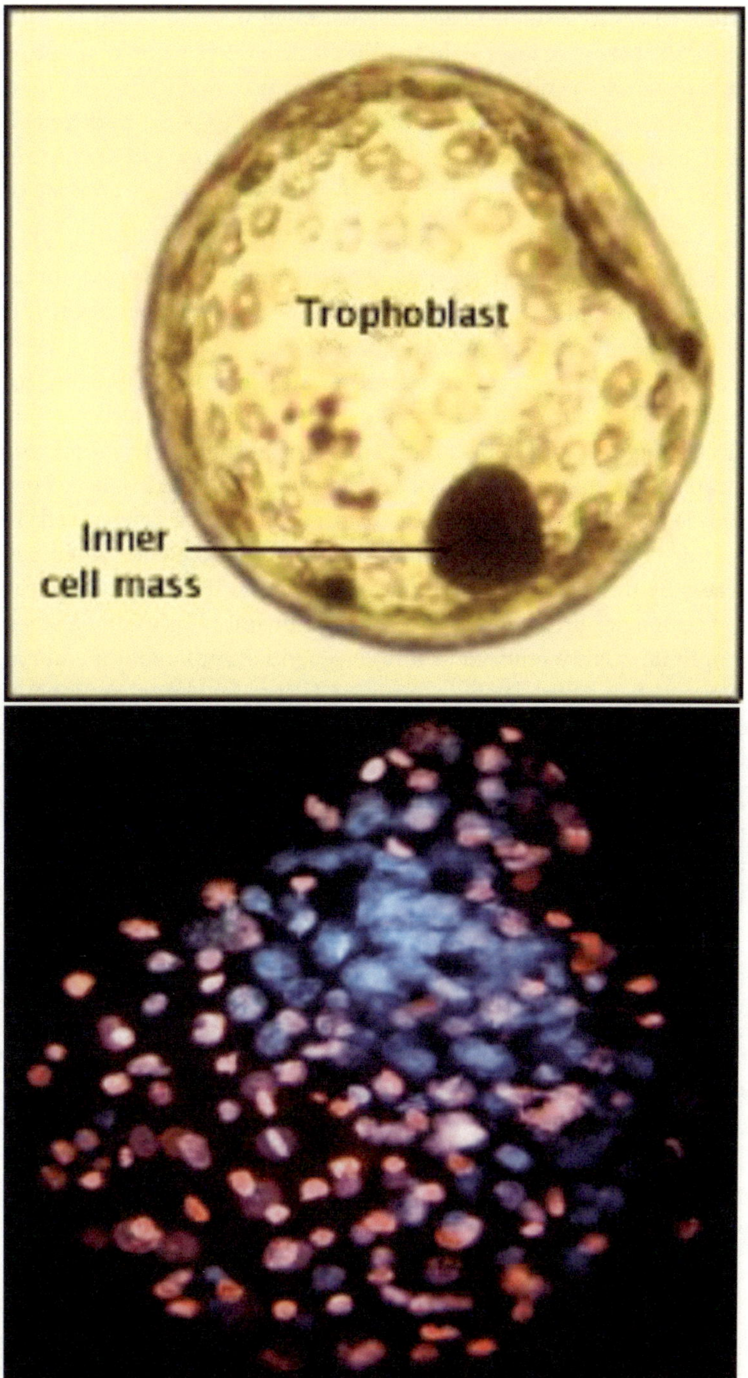

Figure 3. Distinguishing different cells in bovine blastocyst embryos with double staining. Top figure shows a blastocyst embryo with marked inner cell mass (ICM) and around trophectoderm cells (TE). Bottom figure shows double-stained bovine blastocyst embryo with blue as ICM and pink as TE cells. The picture on top is from webpage search, and the author greatly appreciates Prof. Fuliang Du's courtesy for the unpublished bottom photo.

enabled researchers to visualize early development in great detail [3, 4]. Recent light-sheet microscopes use a sheet of laser light to illuminate a thin section of a sample and capture the entire plane in one snapshot. This allows them to use much less light than confocal or two-photon microscopes. It is very fast but also very gentle to perform extremely well in multiple critical ways at the same time [20]. For imaging the development of entire embryos like those of *Drosophila*, zebrafish, and mice, this new multiview imaging technique is fantastic.

Time-lapse imaging is another noninvasive, emerging technology that allows 24-hour monitoring of embryo development, offering the possibility of increased quantity and quality of morphological information without disturbing the culture condition [21]. The time-lapse microscope is very useful for embryo development observation. In the last decade, many human IVF clinics or centers have started to use time-lapse imaging to monitor embryo growth and division during in vitro culture and finally to select good quality embryo for transfer according to record data and pictures. This technique has been reported to be able to improve transferred embryo implantation and pregnancy [22, 23]. Based on time-lapse record for embryo cleavage, normal embryo cleavage speed may be determined. Thus, in the second chapter of this book, the timing of embryo cleavage has been outlined based on morphokinetic markers by the time-lapse monitor. According to this embryo cleavage timing outline, embryologists may clearly know at which stage an embryo should be at various time points. Thus, an optimal quality embryo or a high-potential implantation embryo may be selected for transfer to obtain a higher pregnancy rate. Using time lapse continuously and frequently recording system, some morphokinetic markers can be revealed in time-lapse system. For instance, the rapid division of embryo cells at a given time often results in lower implantation rate. In the normal situation, the division from zygote into 2–3 cells requires about 10–11 hours of time, but Rubio et al. [21] found that some embryos just spend about 5 hours to complete this division, and these embryos have much lower implantation rate than normal division embryos (1.2% vs 20%). Also, embryo unequal cleavage which is defined as an abruption of one blastomere into three daughter blastomeres or an interval of cell cycle less than 5 hours often produces significant lower implantation potential [24]. Thus, we may use these more precise morphokinetic markers to distinguish the embryo quality.

The third chapter further examines and verifies whether time-lapse imaging technology is useful for the selection of "top-quality" embryos for transfer to improve ART outcome rather than conventional morphological evaluation. Interestingly, the possible correlations between the sex of the embryo, embryo fragmentation, treatment protocols, different culture media, and embryo morphokinetics have been evaluated based on some new researches on time-lapse imaging facilities. Furthermore, various algorithms and predictive models designed in ART cycles with time-lapse imaging are also discussed. For example, a lot of researches on animal and human embryonic development speed by ordinary morphology observation showed that male embryos grow faster than female embryos [25–27]. However, current time-lapse imaging observation may provide more detail and exact information on the difference in male and female embryos during early divisions. Although female embryos showed late cleavage (t8), morula (tM), and blastocyst stage morphokinetic parameters, they presented earlier expansion than males. Thus, the key time points of observation is related to embryo gender development. Interestingly, the authors designed a model according to the time of second synchrony and morula formation with four subgroups to predict the probability of an embryo being female.

In order to further study and explore morphokinetics of embryo cleavage, the fourth chapter discusses some methods for **spatiotemporal analysis of embryo cleavage in vitro.** Automated or semiautomated time-lapse analysis of early stage embryo images during the cleavage stage can give insight into the timing of mitosis, regularity of both division timing and pattern, as well as into cell lineage. Simultaneous monitoring of molecular processes enables the study of connections between genetic expression and cell physiology and development. By time-lapse imaging data and analytical software, a four-dimensional video sequencing of embryos can be easily created so that growing embryos display new insights into temporal embryo development. In this chapter, the authors describe three methods with variations in hardware and software analysis by giving some examples of the outcomes to open a window to new information in developmental embryology, as embryo division pattern and lineage are studied in vivo.

2.2. Gene expression of cleavage embryo and noninvasive assessment of embryo viability via culture media analysis

Preimplantation embryo development experiences a series of critical events and remarkable epigenetic modifications, and reprogramming of gene expression occurs to activate the embryonic genome. In the early stages of preimplantation embryo development, maternal mRNAs direct embryonic development. Throughout early embryonic development, a differential methylation pattern is maintained, although some show stage-specific changes. Recent studies have shown that differential demethylation process results in differential parental gene expression in the early developing embryos that may have an impact on the correct development [28]. Also, noncoding RNAs, long noncoding RNAs (lncRNA), and short noncoding RNAs, microRNAs (miRNAs) have been shown to play an important role in the regulation of mRNAs, and therefore their role in preimplantation development has gained significance. Chapter Five reviews the different factors affecting gene expression during preimplantation embryo development, which includes epigenetic factors, focusing on methylation profiles, of gametes and preimplantation embryos. The effects of noncoding RNAs on gene expression were thoroughly evaluated.

Because gene expression appearance during embryo development in in vitro culture, preimplantation embryos often require rich nutrition culture media. The embryo during its growth and development needs to absorb some important nutritive components from culture medium and metabolically produce some by-products as gene expression results. From this point of view, in vitro culturing of embryos also provides a very important material for further noninvasive embryo evaluation by means of examining biomarkers in the spent embryo culture medium. Current developed methods concentrate on the measurement of metabolic compounds secreted from developing embryos. These studies mainly utilize the tools of modern analytics and proteomics. Some studies suggest that metabolic profiling of embryo culture media using optical and nonoptical spectroscopies may provide a useful adjunct to the current embryo assessment strategies and provide insight into the phenotype of embryos with increasing reproductive potential [29].

In the sixth chapter, the authors describe their new discovery, the alpha-1 chain of the human haptoglobin molecule as a quantitative biomarker of embryo viability. In a series of retrospective, blind experiments achieved more than 50% success rate. This chapter summarizes the currently available metabolic and proteomic approaches as the noninvasive molecular assessment of embryo viability. Recent studies showed that the assessment of the molecular components of nutrient media is a promising area in searching for the markers of successful embryo implantation with the subsequent development of a clinical pregnancy and the birth of a healthy baby to enhance the efficiency of treatment using ART techniques [30]. If the molecular composition of cultivation media can be used as an additional noninvasive procedure to choose an embryo for selective transfer, it will be very useful to improve human IVF pregnancy outcome.

3. Improving in vitro culture environment for embryo cleavages

Embryonic quality, cleavage speed, and gene expression have a close relationship with in vitro culture environment, including culture media, incubator type, and gas concentration [31, 32]. Thus, since starting embryo in vitro culture, many studies have concentrated on improving embryo culture condition. For many decades, optimization of culture media for the support of human and animal embryos has been a focus of considerable interest [33]. So far, many commercial embryo culture media are available for human embryo culture, and their effects on embryo culture are varied. The studies comparing these effects of culture media on embryonic development have reported contradictory conclusion. Many studies did not find a significant difference or found just a tiny difference between various culture media [34]. Recently, Mantikou et al. [35] used meta-analysis to evaluate 31 different comparisons for 20 different culture media and could not find which culture medium leads to the best success rates in IVF/ICSI.

Also, incubators in the IVF laboratory play a pivotal role in providing a stable and appropriate culture environment required for optimizing embryo development and clinical outcomes. With technological advances, several types of incubators have been applied to human IVF laboratory. Recently, Swain [32] did a comparative analysis of embryo cultural incubators in human IVF laboratories and reviewed some incubator functions and key environmental variables controlled and the technology utilized in various units. This comparison indicates that smaller benchtop/top-load incubators provide faster recovery of environmental variables, but there is no clear advantage of any particular incubator based on clinical outcomes.

However, based on last decade's IVF practical observation, Dr. Bin Wu's laboratory has found an interesting phenomenon which showed a favorable response of individual patient's embryos to media and incubators. Some patents' embryos grow very well in one kind of medium, but it does not grow well in the other medium. The seventh chapter gives a detailed report on this research result. Thus, in human IVF clinical practice, using two media and two incubators for embryo culture could significantly improve IVF/ICSI embryo quality and increase pregnancy rates.

Author details

Bin Wu

Address all correspondence to: bwu13@yahoo.com

Arizona Center for Reproductive Endocrinology and Infertility, Tucson, Arizona, USA

References

[1] Fragouli E, Alfarawati S, Spath K, Wells D. Morphological and cytogenetic assessment of cleavage and blastocyst stage embryos. Molecular Human Reproduction. 2014;**20** (92):117-126

[2] Kirkegaard K, Ahlstron A, Ingersley HJ, Hardarson T. Choosing the best embryo by time lapse versus standard morphology. Fertility and Sterility. 2015;**103**(2):323-332

[3] Strnad P, Gunther S, Reichmann J, Krzic U, Balazs B, de Medeiros G, Norlin N, Hiiragi T, Hufnagel L, Ellenberg J. Inverted light-sheet microscope for imaging mouse pre-implantation development. Nature Methods. 2015. DOI: 10.1038/nmeth.3690 [Epub ahead of print]

[4] Chhetri RK, Amat F, Wan Y, Höckendorf B, Lemon WC, Keller PJ. Whole-animal functional and developmental imaging with isotropic spatial resolution. Nature Methods. 2015;**12**(12):1171-1178. DOI: 10.1038/nmeth.3632 [Epub: October 26, 2015]

[5] Brachetm A. Recherches sur la de"terminisme he're'ditaire de l'oeuf des mammife'res. De'veloppement in vitro de jeunes ve'sicules blastodermiques de lapin. Archives de Biologie (Lie'ge). 1913;**28**:423-426

[6] Biggers JD. IVF and embryo transfer: Historical origin and development. Fertility Magazine. 2013;**16**:5-15

[7] Whitten WK. Culture of tubal mouse ova. Nature. 1956;**177**(4498):96

[8] Lundin K, Bergh C, Hardarson T. Early embryo cleavage is a strong indicator of embryo quality in human IVF. Human Reproduction. 2001;**16**(2):2652-2657

[9] Payne JF, Raburn DJ, Couchman GM, Price TM, Jamison MG, Walmer DK. Relationship between pre-embryo pronuclear morphology (zygote score) and standard day 2 or 3 embryo morphology with regard to assisted reproductive technique outcomes. Fertility and Sterility. 2005;**84**(4):900-909

[10] Rocowsky C, Vernon M, Mayer J, Ball GD, Behr B, Pomeroy KO, et al. Standardization of grading embryo morphology. Journal of Assisted Reproduction and Genetics. 2010;**27**(8):437-439

[11] Wu B, Tong J, Leibo SP. Effect of cooling germinal vesicle-stage bovine oocytes on meiotic spindle formation following in vitro maturation. Molecular Reproduction and Development. 1999;**54**:388-395

[12] Wu B. Expression of c-fos and c-jun proto-oncogenes by ovine preimplantation embryos. Zygote. 1993;**4**:211-217

[13] Wu B, Ignotz G, Currie WB, Yang X. Dynamics of maturation promoting factor and its constituent proteins during *in vitro* maturation of bovine oocytes. Biology of Reproduction. 1997;**56**:253-259

[14] Wu B, Ignotz G, Currie WB, Yang X. The expression of c-mos proto-oncoprotein in bovine oocytes during maturation *in vitro*. Biology of Reproduction. 1997;**56**:260-265

[15] Puissant F, Rysselberg MV, Barlow P, Deweze J, Leroy F. Embryo scoring as a prognostic tool in IVF treatment. Human Reproduction. 1987;**2**:705

[16] Santos E, Noble J, Wells D. A review on automatic analysis of human embryo microscope image. Open Biomedical Engineering Journal. 2010;**4**:170-177

[17] Molina I, Lazaro-Ibanez E, Pertusa J, Debon A, Martinez-Sanchis JV, Pelicer A. A minimal invasive methodology based on morphometric parameters for day 2 embryo quality assessment. Reproductive BioMedicine Online. 2014;**29**:470-480

[18] Braga DPAF, Setti AS, Figueria RCS, Iaconelli A Jr, Borges E Jr. The importance of the cleavage stage morphology evaluation for blastocyst transfer in patients with good prognosis. Journal of Assisted Reproduction and Genetics. 2014;**31**:1105-1110

[19] Sallam HN, Sallam NH, Sallam SH. Non-invasive methods for embryo selection. Facts, Views & Vision in ObGyn. 2016;**8**(2):87-100

[20] Udan RS, Piazza VG, Hsu CW, Hadjantonakis AK, Dickinson ME. Quantitative imaging of cell dynamics in mouse embryos using light-sheet microscopy. Development. 2014;**141**(22):4406-4414. DOI: 10.1242/dev.111021 [Epub: October 24, 2014]

[21] Rubio I, Kuhlmann R, Agerholm I, Kirk J, Herrero J, Escriba MJ, Bellver J, Meseguer M. Limited implantation success of direct-cleaved human zygotes: A time-lapse study. Fertility and Sterility. 2012;**98**:1458-1463

[22] Meseguer M, Rubio I, Cruz M, Basile N, Marcos J, Requena A. Embryo incubation and selection in a time-lapse monitoring system improves pregnancy outcome compared with a standard incubator: A retrospective cohort study. Fertility and Sterility. 2012;**98**(6):1481-1489.e10

[23] Dominguez F, Meseguer M, Aparicio-Ruiz B, Piqueras P, Quinonero A, Simon C. New strategy for diagnosing embryo implantation potential by combining proteomics and time-lapse technologies. Fertility and Sterility. 2015;**104**(4):908-914

[24] Zhan Q, Ye Z, Clarke R, Rosenwaks Z, Zaninovic N. Direct unequal cleavages: Embryo developmental competence, genetic constitution and clinical outcome. PLoS One. 2016;**11**(12):e0166398. DOI: 10.1371/journal.pone.0166398

[25] Wu B. Amplification of Sry gene allows identification of the sex of mouse preimplantation embryos. Theriogenology. 1993;**40**:441-453

[26] Alfarawati S, Fragouli E, Colls P, Stevens J, Gutierrez-Mateo C, Schoolcraft WB, et al. The relationship between blastocyst morphology, chromosomal abnormality, and embryo gender. Fertility and Sterility. 2011;**95**(2):520-524

[27] Hentemann MA, Briskemyr S, Bertheussen K. Blastocyst transfer and gender: IVF versus ICSI. Journal of Assisted Reproduction and Genetics. 2009;**26**(8):433-436

[28] Oswald J, et al. Active demethylation of the paternal genome in the mouse zygote. Current Biology. 2000;**10**(8):475-478

[29] Botros L, Sakkas D, Seli E. Metabolomics and its application for non-invasive embryo assessment in IVF. Molecular Human Reproduction. 2008;**14**(12):679-690. DOI: 10.1093/molehr/gan066

[30] Zorina IM, Smolnikova VY, Bobrov MY. Study of embryo metabolic products in culture media as a tool for determining the implantation potential. Journal Archive. 2017;**2**:1-6. DOI: 10.18565/aig.2017.2.11-6

[31] Lonergan P, Rizos D, Gutiérrez-Adán A, Fair T, Boland MP. Effect of culture environment on embryo quality and gene expression—experience from animal studies. Reproductive BioMedicine Online. 2003;**7**(6):657-663. Available from: www.rbmonline.com/Article/985 [Accessed: July 23, 2003]

[32] Swain JE. Optimal human embryo culture. Seminars in Reproductive Medicine. 2015;**33**(2):103-117. DOI: 10.1055/s-0035-1546423

[33] Biggers JD. Thoughts on embryo culture conditions. Fertility Magazine. 2014;**16**:34-43

[34] Aoki VW, Wilcox AL, Peterson CM, Parker-Jones K, Hatasaka HH, Huang I, Carrell DT. Comparison of four media types during 3-day human IVF embryo culture. Reproductive BioMedicine Online. 2005;**10**(5):600-606. DOI: 10.1016/S1472-6483(10)61667-7

[35] Mantikou E, Youssef MAFM, van Wely M, van der Veen F, Al-Inany HG, Repping S, Mastenbroek S. Embryo culture media and IVF/ICSI success rates: A systematic review. Human Reproduction Update. 2013;**19**(3):210-220

Section 2

Embryo Cleavage Morphokinetics

Chapter 2

Timing of Embryo Cleavage

Meng Ju Lee

Additional information is available at the end of the chapter

http://dx.doi.org/10.5772/intechopen.69437

Abstract

Time-lapse system can provide a culture environment to observe the development of embryos continuously. There are many morphokinetic markers to help us to find out the best quality of embryos. We review the studies to clarify the relationship of markers between implantation potential and embryo chromosome status. Surprisingly, most of markers are controversial or no significant effect on implantation potential and pregnancy rate. We suppose that some uncertain factors may influence embryonic implantation and pregnancy. Here we provide a new method for selecting optimal quality of embryos by many morphokinetic markers in the time-lapse system. Therefore, we can expect that the time-lapse system helps us to choose the good quality embryos for subsequent embryos transfer to improve implantation potential, euploid chromosome and pregnancy rate. Furthermore, studies need to understand the other maternal physical conditions correlation with embryos implantation.

Keywords: time-lapse, cleavage embryo, morphokinetic markers

1. Introduction

The morphology of embryo is the most widespread method to select the embryo with high implantation potential in assisted reproductive technology (ART). Conventionally, embryo development was daily observed after insemination, which could assist the embryologists to select the optimal embryo to transfer for elevating live birth rate eventually. However, the daily observation is considered as a disadvantage for embryo development because of the frequent transfer between incubator and atmospheric environment. Thus, a new and powerful tool, time-lapse monitor (TLM), was developed to estimate the morphokinetic markers of embryos. Currently, TLM can be used to evaluate the embryo growing status from the time of insemination to blastocyst formation. The sequential assessment of pronuclear, cleavage stage, and blastocyst morphology can continuously evaluate the morphology of embryos through automatically obtaining images in every 5–20 min. Besides, TLM offers a steady culture condition due to bypassing the daily observation. Here, we discuss the timing of embryo cleavage and the following effects of implantation potential in this chapter.

2. Morphokinetic markers

Generally, there are many milestones (**Figure 1**), including pronucleus appearance, pronucleus breakdown, first division, second division and blastulation, during the period of fertilization to blastocyst formation. The TLM fails to obtain the pictures at every minute since the capturing period was limited. Although the limitation of the time lapse is obvious, currently, it is still the most practical manner to evaluate the timing of embryo development rather than daily observation. Here, we listed the morphokinetic markers and discussed the timing of different time point during the development of embryos and the effect of clinical outcomes.

(1) The timing of second polar body extrusion (tPB2): the time of the second polar body extrusion is 2.9 ± 0.1 h after Intra-cytoplasmic sperm injection (ICSI). The range of extrusion time is around 0.7–10.15 h. If the oocytes from female age >38 years old, the timing of second polar body extrusion was significantly delayed but no other effects were observed in further embryo development [1]. The mean time of tPB2 is 3.9 h in euploid and 4.0 h in aneuploid embryos, respectively. The chromosome integrity of embryos is irrelevant to the timing of second body extrusion [2].

(2) The timing of pronuclear appearance (tPNa): the time of pronuclear appearance is 8.4 ± 2.4 h in the implantation group and 8.2 ± 1.9 h in the non-implantation group [3]. In euploid embryos, the mean time of tPNa is 10.2 h and 10.1 h in aneuploid embryos [2]. Therefore, the timing of pronuclear appearance has no significant effect on implantation potential and chromosome status.

(3) The timing of pronuclear fading (tPNf): longer time taken in pronucleus (PN) breakdown might be beneficial for live birth. Azzarello et al. [4] claimed that the timing of tPNf was longer in live birth group (24.9 ± 0.6 vs. 23.3 ± 0.4 h), and there was no live birth if the timing of PN breakdown was less than 20 h. The timing of PN breakdown was equal between implanted and non-implanted embryos [3, 5]. The mean time of tPNf is 24.4 h in euploid embryos and 24.8 h in aneuploid embryos [2]. The timing of pronuclear fading has no significant difference in embryo implantation and chromosome status but no live birth when tPNf is less than 20 h.

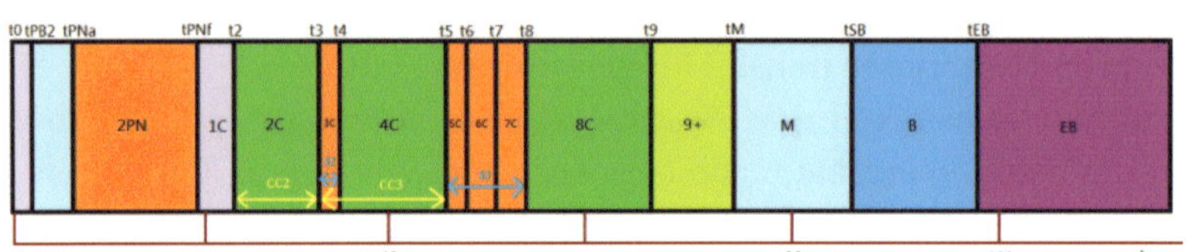

Figure 1. The milestones of embryo development. tPB2: the timing of second polar body extrusion, tPNa: the timing of pronuclear appearance, tPNf: the timing of pronuclear fading, t2, 3, 4, 5, 6, 7, 8, 9: time from insemination to the 2, 3, 4, 5, 6, 7, 8, 9 cell stages, tM: time from insemination to morula, tSB: time from insemination to starting blastulation, tEB: time from insemination to expanded blastulation, cc2:t3-t2, cc3:t5-t3, s2:t4-t3, s3:t8-t5.

(4) Time from insemination to the 2-cell stage (t2): it is still controversial in the period. Meseguer et al. [6] presented that the t2 of implanted embryos group was shorter than non-implanted embryos (25.6 ± 2.2 vs. 26.7 ± 3.8 h). Chamayou et al. [3] showed no significant difference in implanted and non-implanted embryos (26.9 ± 3.2 vs. 27.0 ± 4.0 h). Kirkegaard et al. [5] claimed that t2 was similar in the pregnancy and non-pregnant groups. Curiously, t2 is shorter when embryo was incubated in single culture medium than sequential culture medium (27.36 ± 4.12 vs. 29.09 ± 4.86 h) [7]. The mean time of t2 is no significant between euploid (28 h) and aneuploid embryos (28.4 h) [2]. The development of the 2-cell stage may be faster in implanted embryos but no significant in chromosome status.

(5) Time from insemination to the 3, 4, 5 cells (t3, t4, t5): some studies have shown that the enhanced implantation potential has been observed in shorter t3, t4 and t5. The time periods of t3, t4 and t5 were significantly shorter in implanted embryos than non-implanted embryos. The times of t3 (37.4 ± 2.8 h), t4 (38.2 ± 3.0 h) and t5 (52.3 ± 4.2 h) are significant difference in implanted embryos compared with the times of t3 (38.4 ± 5.2 h), t4 (40.0 ± 5.4 h) and t5 (52.6 ± 6.8 h) in non-implanted embryos [6]. However, Chamayou et al. [3] and Kirkegaard et al. [5] demonstrated that there was no difference in embryo implantation and pregnancy rate. The embryo development is faster in single culture medium than in sequential culture medium (t3, 37.75 ± 6.64 vs. 39.53 ± 6.15 h; t4, 40.07 ± 5.98 vs. 41.45 ± 6.07 h; t5, 48.77 ± 9.49 vs. 52.22 ± 9.34 h) [7]. The mean time of t3 (37.4 vs. 37.2 h) and t5 (50.4 vs. 50.6 h) is no significant difference between euploid and aneuploid embryos, but the mean time of t4 (40 h) is significant difference between the euploid (40 h) and aneuploidy (41.1 h) blastocysts [2]. Consequently, faster embryo development of t3, 4, 5 is beneficial for implantation, but only t4 might influence the euploid rate of blastocysts.

(6) Time from insemination to the 6, 7, 8, 9 cells (t6, t7, t8, t9): according to the previous report, although the time from insemination to the 8 cells exhibited faster in implanted embryos (54.9 ± 5.2 vs. 58.0 ± 7.2 h) [8], the other report showed that there are no statistical difference between the implanted and nonimplanted embryos at t6 (54.3 ± 5.8 vs. 54.5 ± 8.2 h), t7 (57.4 ± 8.6 vs. 57.6 ± 9.8 h), t8 (61.0 ± 10.8 vs. 60.8 ± 11.5 h) and t9 (77 ± 8.5 vs. 76 ± 11.3 h) [3]. In addition, Kirkegaard et al. [5] also proved that the pregnant rate was irrelevant to the period. In euploid embryos, the t6 (53.9 h), t7 (57.8 h), t8 (61.9 h) and t9 (76.1 h) are similar to the time in aneuploid embryos [2]. Statistically, the t6, t7, t8 and t9 have no significant difference between the implanted and non-implanted embryos and between the euploid and aneuploid embryos.

(7) Time from insemination to morula (tM): morula is defined as all cells fused together. There is no difference that the tM is 86 ± 9.1 and 84.4 ± 11.4 h in implanted and non-implanted embryos, respectively [3]. The tM of euploid (94.4 h) and aneuploid (95.3 h) are insignificant [2]. Therefore, statistically, the tM does not involve in the implantation potential and chromosome status.

(8) Time from insemination to starting blastulation (tSB): the initiation of blastulation means the time point of the blastocoel cavity observation. There is no significant difference in the mean time of tSB in implantation and pregnancy [3, 5]. Therefore, the time from insemination to starting blastulation does not affect embryo implantation potential and pregnancy rate. However, the mean time of tSB (103.4 h) in euploid embryos is significant shorter than

aneuploid embryos (103.4 h, $p = 0.007$) [2]. Furthermore, the shorter tSB refers to more chance of euploid embryos for embryo transfer.

(9) Time period from insemination to expanded blastulation (tEB): expanded blastulation means the diameter of blastocyst had increased by more than 30%, the expanding results in a thin zona pellucida [9]. There is no *statistical significance* between implanted embryos and non-implanted embryos (111.7 vs. 110.5 h) [3]. Kirkegaard et al. [5] also indicated that there is no significant difference in pregnancy and non-pregnancy groups (104 h). However, the mean time of tEB is significant shorter in euploid embryos than that in aneuploid embryos (118.7 vs. 122.1 h) [2]. In addition, the shorter time of embryos achieved expanded blastulation is more likely to be euploid embryo. The faster embryos of expanded blastulation have more euploid embryos but the meant time of tEB has no difference between implantation potential and pregnancy.

(10) Time period between 2-cell and 3-cell stage (t3-t2, cc2): cleavage cycle 2, time of the second cycle is also known as the time between 2-cell and 3-cell stage. The mean of cc2 is 11.4 h in implanted embryos and 11.8 h in non-implanted embryos [3]. Meseguer et al. [6] found the same cc2 (11.8 h) in implanted and non-implanted embryos. The mean of cc2 (11 h) is also no *statistical significance* between pregnancy and non-pregnancy group [5]. There is no difference in the mean of cc2 in euploid and aneuploid embryos (10.5 vs. 10.4 h) [2]. Therefore, cc2 cannot predict the implantation potential, pregnancy rate and chromosome status.

(11) Time period between 5-cell and 3-cell stages (t5-t3, cc3): it is also defined as cleavage cycle 3 by Chamayou et al. [3]. They presented that the median of cc3 was significant longer in implanted embryos than nonimplanted embryos (14.4 and 13.0 h, respectively). As a result, longer cc3 may be beneficial for embryo development.

(12) Time of synchrony of the second cell cycle (s2, t4-t3): time between 4-cell and 3-cell stages or 3-cell stage also means s2. The mean of s2 is 2 h in implanted embryos and 1.7 h in non-implanted embryos [3]. It also has no significant difference between pregnancy and non-pregnancy groups [5]. However, the mean of s2 is significant smaller in euploid embryos than aneuploid embryos (2.6 vs. 4.2 h) [2]. Therefore, the mean of s2 might be used for predicting the chromosome status of embryos.

(13) Time of synchrony of the third cell cycle (s3, t8-t5): S3 also signifies the time between 8-cell and 5-cell stages. It includes the sum of 5-cell, 6-cell and 7-cell stages. There is no difference in the mean of s3 between implanted embryos and non-implanted embryos (8.0 vs. 8.1 h) [3]. Kirkegaard et al. [5] also found no difference between pregnancy and non-pregnancy groups. There are no data compared with the mean of s3 in aneuploid and non-aneuploid embryos. Hence, the effect of s3 on implanted potential and pregnancy rate remains no significantly.

3. Special markers in time-lapse system

Some morphokinetic markers are only revealed in the time-lapse system because the continuously and frequently recording system. Traditional observation has difficulty in observing these transitory phenomena. Following this, we listed these morphokinetic markers and conclude the effect of embryos.

Direct cleavage (≦5 h from 2 to 3 cells): generally, the time from 2 to 3 cells is around 10–11 h [2, 3, 5, 6]. Rubio et al. [10] found that embryos with direct cleavage (≦5 h) have lower implantation rate than embryos with normal cleavage pattern (1.2 vs. 20%). The incidence rate of direct cleavage is 14%. What is the reason causing direct cleavage is still obscure. Based on the announcement of Rubio et al. [10], the centrioles introduced by the sperm control the first mitotic divisions of the oocytes. Therefore, the impairment of sperm neck, the location of centrioles, during ICSI procedure may alter the timing of first embryos cleavage. Rejection of direct cleavage embryos for transfer could enhance the implantation rate.

Direct unequal cleavage (DUC): actually, direct cleavage could occur at any cleavage cycle. Zhan et al. [11] defined as the abrupt cleavage of one blastomere into three daughter blastomeres or an interval of cell cycles less than 5 h. Therefore, they describe direct unequal cleavage at first cleavage as DUC-1, at second cleavage as DUC-2, at third cleavage as DUC-3 and embryos exhibiting multiple DUCs as DUC-Plus. They found that the embryos fertilized with the sperm from epididymis, and testicles have significant higher DUP-1 percentage (13.6 vs. 11.4%). However, the incidence of DUS-1 is 9.1% in embryos fertilized with sperm from ejaculation. Besides, the embryos with multinucleation blastomere (MNB) have 2–3 times of incidence compared to non-MNB embryos. They conclude that blastocyst rate, implantation potential and euploid rate are significantly lower in DUC embryos. Non-DUC embryos should be the first choice for embryos transfer.

Reverse cleavage: reverse cleavage can be divided into two types. Reverse cleavage type 1 (complete): blastomeres rejoin after completely separating. Reverse cleavage type 2 (incomplete): zygote or blastomere fails to separate (type I, Supplemental Video 1; type 2, Supplemental Videos 2 are available online at www.fertstert.org). It could occur up to three times in 27.4% of embryos during the first three cleavage cycles [12]. They found GnRH antagonist protocol and ICSI procedure had higher incidence of reverse cleavage compared with GnRH agonist protocol and IVF procedure. Embryos fertilizing with poor sperm motility (<21%) also have higher rate of reverse cleavage. Besides, embryos with reverse cleavage are associated with poor grade embryos and lower implantation potential. Therefore, reverse cleavage is a negative factor for embryos selection.

4. Conclusion

The continuously morphokinetic change of embryo development is the main characteristic of time-lapse system. We can observe many milestones of embryos development and calculate the time intervals to understand the relationship of implantation potential, chromosome status and pregnancy rate. Unfortunately, all the morphokinetic markers could not predict implantation potential, chromosome status and pregnancy rate exactly. Most of markers are controversial or no significant effect. Conventionally, embryos with quicker development would be recommended for transfer to raise the pregnancy rate. However, after reviewing all the data, not all markers can support this principle.

The reason of controversial descriptions of the markers is very incomprehensive. We suppose that some factors might influence embryos implantation and pregnancy. Obviously, maternal and physical conditions, such as endometrial receptivity, endometrial polyps, endometrial or endocervical infection, hydrosalpinx, immune disorder, subclinical hypothyroidism etc., can also impede the embryos implantation and the following pregnancy. We also know that aneuploid embryos show poor implantation rate or result in spontaneous abortion. Although some markers correlate with higher rate of euploid embryos, it still cannot be used for predicting euploid embryos precisely. If people want to know the chromosome status of embryos, pre-implantation genetic screening (PGS) is still the first choice.

Therefore, the time-lapse system can help us to evaluate the quality of embryos. We can use more precise morphokinetic markers to distinguish the embryos quality. The embryos with good quality have higher rate of implantation potential and normal chromosome. Currently, PGS is the optimal manner to find out the euploid embryos. However, the good quality of euploid embryo is not a guarantee of embryo implantation and pregnancy. It is the basic condition for better embryo implantation. We have to consider many other maternal and physical situations which greatly affect embryo implantation to promote the implantation and pregnancy rate. It also needs further studies to clarify the mystery of implantation process.

Author details

Meng Ju Lee

Address all correspondence to: swrh1214@gmail.com

Stork Fertility Center, Stork Ladies Clinic, Hsinchu, Taiwan

References

[1] Liu Y, Chapple V, Roberts P, Ali J, Matson P. Time-lapse videography of human oocytes following intracytoplasmic sperm injection: Events up to the first cleavage division. Reproductive Biology. 2014;**14**(4):249-256

[2] Minasi MG, Colasante A, Riccio T, Ruberti A, Casciani V, Scarselli F, Spinella F, Fiorentino F, Varricchio MT, Greco E. Correlation between aneuploidy, standard morphology evaluation and morphokinetic development in 1730 biopsied blastocysts: A consecutive case series study. Human Reproduction. 2016;31(10):2245-2254

[3] Chamayou S, Patrizio P, Storaci G, Tomaselli V, Alecci C, Ragolia C, Crescenzo C, Guglielmino A. The use of morphokinetic parameters to select all embryos with full capacity to implant. Journal of Assisted Reproduction and Genetics. 2013;30:703-710

[4] Azzarello A, Hoest T, Mikkelsen AL. The impact of pronuclei morphology and dynamicity on live birth outcome after time-lapse culture. Human Reproduction. 2012;27:2649-2657

[5] Kirkegaard K, Kesmodel US, Hindkjaer JJ, Ingerslev HJ. Time-lapse parameters as predictors of blastocyst development and pregnancy outcome in embryos from good prognosis patients: A prospective cohort study. Human Reproduction. 2013;**28**(10):2643-2651

[6] Meseguer M, Herrero J, Tejera A, Hilligsoe KM, Ramsing NB, Remohi J. The use of morphokinetic as a predictor of embryo implantation. Human Reproduction. 2011;**26**:2658-2671

[7] Ciray HN, Aksoy T, Goktas C, Ozturk B, Bahceci M. Time-lapse evaluation of human embryo development in single versus sequential culture media—A sibling oocyte study. Journal of Assisted Reproduction and Genetics. 2012;29(9):891-900

[8] Dal Canto M, Coticchio G, RenziniMM, DePonti E, Novara PV, Brambillasca F, Comi R, Fadini R. Cleavage kinetics analysis of human embryos predicts development to blastocyst and implantation. Reproductive Biomedicine Online. 2012;**25**:474-480

[9] Campbell A, Fishel S, Bowman N, Duffy S, Sedler M, Hickman CFL. Modelling a risk classification of aneuploidy in human embryos using non-invasive morphokinetics. Reproductive Biomedicine Online. 2013;**26**:477-485

[10] Rubio I, Kuhlmann R, Agerholm I, Kirk J, Herrero J, Escriba MJ, Bellver J, Meseguer M. Limited implantation success of direct-cleaved human zygotes: A time-lapse study. Fertility and Sterility. 2012;**98**:1458-1463

[11] Zhan Q, Ye Z, Clarke R, Rosenwaks Z, Zaninovic N. Direct unequal cleavages: Embryo developmental competence, genetic constitution and clinical outcome. PLoS ONE. 2016;**11**(12):e0166398. DOI:10.1371/journal. pone.0166398

[12] Liu Y, Chapple V, Roberts P, Matson P. Prevalence, consequence, and significance of reverse cleavage by human embryos viewed with the use of the Embryoscope time-lapse video system. Fertility and Sterility. 2014;**102**:1295-1300

Chapter 3

Embryo Morphokinetics Based on Time-Lapse Observation

Nasim Tabibnejad

Additional information is available at the end of the chapter

http://dx.doi.org/10.5772/intechopen.69226

Abstract

Embryo incubation and evaluation are critical steps in assisted reproductive technology (ART). Conventionally, embryo assessment has been done by embryologists through removing embryos from a conventional incubator during the culture period. Over recent years, time-lapse systems (TLS) have been established which can take digital images of embryos at key points and time intervals. This technique allows embryologists to assess the embryo quality in the steady culture environment. According to TLS studies and prepared algorithm models, it seems that TLS alone or in combination with conventional morphology can be considered as a useful diagnostic tool to determine high-quality embryos and improve embryonic implantation and pregnancy rates. In addition, there were remarkable differences between embryo developmental time points and intervals regarding embryo gender, embryo fragmentation, and type of ovarian stimulation protocol. For confident conclusion, time-lapse imaging should be evaluated in further studies, and the system should be evaluated for cost/benefit ratio effectiveness in individual laboratory.

Keywords: embryo cleavage, embryo morphokinetics, embryoscope, time-lapse imaging

1. Introduction

Assisted reproductive technology (ART) may help infertile couples to realize their dream to have a child in their family, but pregnancy and live birth rates following in vitro fertilization (IVF) still remain low. It is ideal to identify viable embryos with the highest implantation potential to raise IVF success rates. In the traditional IVF practice, embryo assessments are mainly based on the morphologic observation and grade of embryologists at each stage of oocyte and embryonic development. Some features including oocyte and embryo quality, blastomere numbers and regularity, the percentage of fragmentation, and cytoplasmic granularity have been defined as prognostic indicators of successful pregnancy. This traditional embryo assessment method may have some detrimental effects on embryo growth because frequently opening and closing of incubators often cause to the change of embryo culture environmental steadiness. In order to reduce the inter- and intra-observer difference change, the time-lapse imaging (TLI) has been introduced into in vitro fertilization (IVF) laboratory. The application of time-lapse technology to the clinical IVF laboratory has supported more detailed observations on the embryo development researches quickly.

The aim of this chapter is to determine whether TLI is useful for selection of "top quality" embryos for transfer to improve ART outcome rather than conventional morphological evaluation. The possible correlation between embryos' sex, embryo fragmentation, treatment protocols, different culture media, and embryo morphokinetics will be examined based on some new researches of TLI facilities. Furthermore, various algorithms and predictive models designed in ART cycles with TLI will be discussed.

2. Time-lapse monitoring system

The main goal in ART procedure is to improve transferred embryo implantation rate and pregnancy outcome which is influenced by many factors. A major question is how to observe embryo growth and development in in vitro culture system. Recently, a new embryo culture system with time-lapse imaging has started to be used in human IVF laboratory practice. In this automating embryology, crucial events during embryo cleavage can be monitored without removing embryo from the incubator. This technique application may protect embryos from environmental variations in temperature, pH, and humidity during embryo culture. On the other hand, the time-lapse systems (TLS) application may reduce the errors of embryo assessment which depends on embryologist's expertise and capabilities. With continuous image recording, some key events during embryo development might be recorded more completely for embryo evaluation. Another problem fronting IVF is multiple pregnancies which increased maternal and fetal complications. Worldwide, many human IVF centers or clinics tend to decrease the number of transferred embryo by elective single-embryo transfer (eSET) based on selecting high potential embryo for transfer. Time-lapse photography can help embryologist choose the most viable embryo and reduce multiple pregnancy rate. The application of TLI was initially demonstrated by Wong et al. who revealed that primary cell divisions can be considered as a tool for embryo assessment and prediction of embryo development [1]. Next, Meseguer et al. reported the association of early cleavage division timing and intervals with embryo ability for implantation [2]. Time-lapse imaging carries a noninvasive alternative to the traditional embryo morphologic assessment using developmental kinetics as well as embryo morphology and accurate observation of cellular uncommon events, such as direct cleavage to three cells, blastomere fusion, multinucleation, and fragment reabsorption [3].

http://dx.doi.org/10.5772/intechopen.69226

2.1. Time-lapse morphokinetic parameters and embryo pregnancy potential

2.1.1. Arguments supporting predictive value of TLS

Embryo assessment by TLS combined with conventional morphologic observation may improve implantation and pregnancy rate. Adamson et al. studied 319 embryo transfer cycles which were divided to standard morphology alone and TLS and morphologic evaluation (case group). The results showed that implantation rate was 30.2 versus 19.0%, and clinical pregnancy rate was 46.0 versus 32.1%, in case and control groups, respectively ($P < 0.05$) [4]. In a historical cohort study, it is indicated that three embryo morphokinetics in the first 48 hours of culture including short duration of the first cytokinesis, duration of the three-cell stage, and absence of direct cleavage to three cells are associated with developing embryos to high-quality blastocysts [5]. Milewski et al. also analyzed developmental data of 1060 embryos and claimed that embryo morphokinetic parameters are related to reaching blastocyst stage and implantation capability and can be reflected in embryo quality. The most different morphokinetic parameters were median of t9 (the time from insemination to the ninth division), t8_int (the stage after the third division), and cc4 (the fourth round of cleavage) between the groups with and without chemical and clinical pregnancy [6]. In a randomized, double-blinded, controlled trial, 930 patients were divided randomly into two groups. A total of 2638 embryos monitored by TLS in case group and 2427 embryos cultured in standard incubator are considered as controls. Implantation rate (44.9 versus 37.1%) and ongoing pregnancy rate (51.4 versus 41.7%) were significantly higher in embryos monitored with TLS compared to control group, respectively. It is also reported that early pregnancy loss was meaningfully reduced in TL-monitored embryos (16.6%) compared to standard-cultured embryos (25.8%) [7]. A total of 648 embryos, resulting from 60 patients, were prospectively evaluated during culture in TLS. The embryos are cultured until Day 5 (blastocyst stage). Early cleavage division time (t2, t4, and t8) and morula (tMor), start of blastulation (tSB), blastocyst (tBL), and expanded blastocyst (tEBL) were remarkably higher in discarded embryos in comparison to blastocysts. Also, early embryo kinetic parameters are correlated to the implantation potential, but this correlation was not observed in late embryo kinetic parameters [8]. Moreover, in a prospective multicenter cohort study, 1727 embryos were evaluated in 5 IVF centers using TL monitoring in combination with Early Embryo Viability Assessment (Eeva). The main outcome was the evaluation of embryologists' skill to choose embryos using Day-3 morphology alone compared to application of both morphology and Eeva. The reported specificities for three embryologists who used morphology or morphology plus Eeva were 59.7 versus 86.3%, 41.9 versus 84.0%, and 79.5 versus 86.6%, respectively. Results showed that using Eeva in combination with Day-3 morphology significantly upgraded experienced embryologists' capability to recognize embryos which may extend to the blastocyst stage [9]. In consistence, another study used the aforementioned methodology with five embryologists and found similar results. The odds ratio by using only morphology assessment was 1.68 (95% CI = 1.29–2.19), while conventional morphology in combination with Eeva Test resulted in higher odds ratio for predicting blastocyst formation 2.57 (95% CI = 1.88–3.51). Therefore, addition of the Eeva Test to traditional embryo evaluation decreased the inconsistency among embryologists [10]. Furthermore, in a large cohort study, 9530 embryos inseminated by intracytoplasmic sperm injection (ICSI) were cultured in TL incubator. Cases were evaluated in four subgroups including "regular divisions," "viable eight cells," "viable blastocyst," and "implanted embryos." Significant differences were reported between "regular divisions" and "viable eight cells" regarding for t2, t3, t5, cc2, cc3, s2, and s3. The timing of t5, t8, tM, cc3, and s2 was remarkably higher in "viable blastocyst" compared to the "viable eight-cell" group. Implanted embryos showed a higher rate for time of t8, tM, tB, and s2 when equated to blastocysts. The results confirmed TLS accuracy for detecting embryo development and implantation potential [11]. Similarly, in an observational study with large sample size, 7483 zygotes inseminated by ICSI were cultured in TLS. Seventeen morphokinetic parameters were evaluated, and a number of significant correlations were found between them and both blastocyst formation and implantation. The most prognostic parameters for blastocyst formation included time of morula formation (tM) and t8–t5. These parameters were less predictive for implantation potential. The parameters with the power of implantation prediction were time for expansion blastocyst (tEB) and t8–t5 [12].

2.1.2. *Arguments against predictive value of TLS*

In a randomized controlled trial, Park et al. compared 240 patients in a closed culture time-lapse system (TLS) with 124 patients in conventional incubator. They reported no significant differences in the number of four-cell embryos, implantation, and ongoing pregnancy rates. They also found a significant higher miscarriage rate in the TLS group [13]. These results are in line with other studies, which showed similar results in good quality embryos, embryo development, blastocyst rate, implantation, and ongoing pregnancy rates between customary culture and TLS [14–16]. In the same way, in a two-part study, poor-prognosis patients have shown no differences in Day-3 embryo quality, implantation, and clinical pregnancy rates between embryos cultured in EmbryoScope™ and conventional culture, whereas in the second portion, embryos developed in the EmbryoScope™ revealed significantly poorer quality on Day 3 compared to standard-cultured embryos [17]. Likewise, in a recent study, a total of 2092 embryos undergoing IVF cycles were evaluated by conventional morphology assessment or TLS. As results indicated, clinical pregnancy rate with transfer of Day-5 embryos was three times higher than Day-3 transfer. But clinical pregnancy rate (68 versus 63%) and implantation rate (51 versus 45%) were comparable between conventional and TLS groups, respectively [18].

In summary, new indicators based on timings and the appearance of abnormal morphological events can only be identified through time-lapse technology. Most of these markers which are detected during the early developmental embryo stages provide early and effective decision regarding embryo selection. Furthermore, it appears that kinetic parameters observed by TLS can predict blastocyst formation with high development ability. However, more studies including accurate meta-analysis should be performed to aid embryologists select embryos with high implantation potential.

2.2. Effect of gender status on embryo morphokinetics

There is a hypothesis that embryo developmental stages are different between male and female embryos and it is showed in animal studies [19, 20]. For human embryos, it is reported that male embryos grow faster than females [21, 22] but other studies negate this theory [23, 24]. Nowadays, developing of TLS for observing embryo developmental process allows monitoring embryos exactly during early divisions. A number of 78 female and 60 male embryos were observed retrospectively. Embryos were cultured in TLS with 100% implantation and identified gender status. As results, female embryos presented earlier expansion than males. But the other key time points and intervals were as the same as blastocyst rate formation [23]. Similarly, 81 live births from successfully treated ART cycles evaluated, respectively. Results indicated that female status is related to late cleavage (t8), morula (tM), and blastocyst-stage morphokinetic parameters. The authors concluded that some expanded blastocyst-stage morphokinetic variables are correlated with female embryo gender [25]. Otherwise, in another study 176 male and 161 female embryos were evaluated, and there were remarkable differences between embryo developmental time points and intervals regarding gender. The authors designed a model according to the time of second synchrony and morula formation with four subgroups to predict the probability of an embryo being female [26]. It seems that further studies with larger samples are needed to confirm the association between embryo morphokinetics and gender status.

2.3. Fragmentation impact on embryo morphokinetics

Fragmentation is a common pattern in early embryo development stages. In conventional morphological embryo assessment, high fragmented embryos are considered inappropriate for transfer or cryopreservation due to low implantation potential [27]. An increase and decrease in the number and volume of fragments as well as reabsorption and lysis may take place during the embryo culture period, and these events could not be detected without using time-lapse system. Application of time-lapse incubator and embryoscope in recent years provides an opportunity to get more information of embryonic growth at different time points rather than morphologic evaluation at particular time point. Stensen et al. evaluated 1943 oocytes and 372 embryos using the PolScope instrument and TL imaging, respectively. It is reported that embryos with <10% fragmentation (low degree) at 42–45 hours after insemination were originated from oocytes with an early presence of the meiotic spindle, quick first mitosis, late start of the second mitosis, and a smaller period of the third mitosis. However, embryos with high fragmentation (>50% fragmentation) were resulted from oocytes with late appearance of meiotic spindle (36.5 hours after human chorionic gonadotropin (hCG) injection), delayed start of the first mitosis (29.8 hours after insemination), early initiation of the second mitosis (36.4 hours after insemination), and a longer interval of the third mitotic cell cycle [28]. It is reported before that fragmentation during early embryo developmental stages is related to mitotic errors [27]. In Stensen's study, it is confirmed that highly fragmented embryos at the time of the first mitotic cell division could not reabsorb fragmentation and considered as embryos with the high level of fragmentation during morphological assessment. According to the aforementioned data, a correlation was noticed between fragmentation and progress of the meiotic and the mitotic cell cycles among in vitro-derived embryos.

2.4. Effect of ovarian stimulation protocol on embryo morphokinetics

The quality of oocytes and embryos is affected by several factors in in vitro cycles. One of these elements is treatment protocol which is applied for ovarian stimulation in ART cycles and is dependent to patient's condition and clinician's decision. It is confirmed that gonadotropin type which is used for ovarian control, increase hormone levels in follicular fluid as well as apoptosis in cumulus cells [29]. Recently, the effect of different drugs and dosage used in ovarian stimulation on embryo quality has been evaluating via TLS. Munoz and colleagues monitored 2817 embryos in oocyte donation cycles by TLS retrospectively. They reported that embryos derived from cycles stimulated by gonadotropin-releasing hormone (GnRH) antagonist + GnRH agonist divided faster than embryos originated from patients who treated with GnRH agonist + human chorionic gonadotropin (hCG). But the difference was not significant between groups excluding the first developmental stage [30]. In addition, the other retrospective study examined 739 embryos by TLS and compared the embryo morphokinetics among patients who triggered by hCG versus GnRHa using TLS. They found developmental delay in embryos originated from hCG-triggered cycles compared to embryos derived from cycles triggered by GnRHa [31]. Conversely, there was no significant difference between three studied groups by TLS regarding embryo morphokinetics. The patients were treated with only recombinant Follicle-stimulating hormone (rFSH), only human menopausal gonadotropin (HMG), and a combination of FSH and HMG. The time points and time intervals in rFSH group reported close-to-ideal timing with no significant difference [32]. According to limited mentioned studies, it can be concluded that the type of ovarian stimulation protocol affects embryo developmental kinetics in different patterns.

2.5. Effect of the type of culture media on embryo morphokinetics

It is proven that culture media components and conditions are important for optimal embryo development. These days the effect of culture media on embryo morphokinetics is visible accurately by using TL monitoring system. Animal research using TLS confirmed the effect of different culture media with varied components on blastocyst formation [33]. In a cohort study, 532 human embryos were cultured in 2 different media, Global as single-step medium and Sage Cleavage as sequential medium. Embryos are monitored by TLS regarding two cells (t2), three cells (t3), four cells (t4), and five cells (t5) as the same as the length of the second cell cycle (cc2) and the synchrony in the division from two to four cells (s2). There were no significant differences between embryos regarding mentioned time points between two culture media. The implantation and pregnancy rates were comparable between groups [34]. The results of a randomized clinical trial on 1356 embryos were similar to the mentioned study. All zygotes were divided into two single steps and sequential media randomly and monitored in TLS until Day 5. The percentages of good quality blastocyst on Day 5 were equivalent between two groups. However, the number of good quality embryos on Day 3 was significantly higher among embryos cultured in single-step medium. Eleven morphokinetic parameters were evaluated, and only four parameters (t7, t8, t3c4c—time between the first observation of 3 and 4 completely separated blastomeres, and t5c7c—time between the first observation of 5 and 7 completely separated blastomeres) differ significantly between embryos cultured in altered media. The authors concluded that single-step culture medium is as nutrient as sequential media for blastocyst development [35]. Costa-Borges et al. compared embryo morphokinetics in single culture media with and without medium renewal on Day 3 of culture. The results revealed no significant differences in good quality blastocysts, blastocyst formation rate, embryo early and late morphokinetics as well as clinical pregnancy, take-home baby rate, and perinatal outcomes [36].

According to the restricted mentioned study, it seems that single-step and sequential media have equivalent effect on embryo morphokinetics. However, additional researches are needed for confirmation of this theory.

2.6. Morphokinetic algorithms for prediction of embryo implantation potential

Developing of TLS provides the opportunity to observe continuous embryo development. Embryologists can select the most viable embryo using a new scoring system based on embryo morphokinetics. It seems that a globally accepted algorithm is needed to predict embryo implantation potential. For the first time, Meseguer et al. introduced a hierarchical model using early embryo morphokinetics. They divided 247 evaluated embryos to 6 subsections, and 4 of these groups were further subdivided into two subcategories. Based on the findings, the multivariable model was designed to categorize embryos according to their implantation potential [37]. Four years later validation of this model was evaluated in a retrospective study by Freour et al. They calculated the implantation rate matching to each subgroup designed by Meseguer's model and analyzed the same data in subgroups according to the day of embryo transfer. The findings did not show the same sensitivity of Meseguer's model for prediction of implantation rate according to morphokinetic subgroups [38]. For creating a time-lapse deselecting model, 270 embryos transferred on Day 3 with known implantation data (KID) were analyzed based on both qualitative and quantitative parameters retrospectively. In addition, 66 KID embryos were evaluated subsequently for validation of the model. Qualitative deselection parameters were described as poor conventional morphology on Day 3, abnormal cleavage patterns detected by time-lapse monitoring, and less than eight cells at 68 hours post-insemination. Quantitative parameters were the time from pronuclear fading (PNF) to five-cell stage and duration of three-cell stage. In conclusion this deselecting method reported as a reliable tool for embryo selection [39]. In a retrospective multicentric study, 1664 intracytoplasmic sperm injection (ICSI) cycles were analyzed. Of them 799 were used to generate an algorithm, and 865 cycles were applied to exam its predictive value in the second study phase. The timing to two cells (t2), three cells (t3), four cells (t4), and five cells (t5) as well as the length of the second cell cycle (cc2 = t3−t2) and the synchrony in the division from two to four cells (s2 = t4−t3) were studied, and both implantation and clinical pregnancy rates were investigated. Three parameters of t3, cc2, and t5 are related to implantation. According to these data, embryos were categorized to four subgroups. In the second phase of the study, the algorithm was authenticated among 1620 transferred embryos. In this phase, embryos were classified based on the algorithm, and significant differences in implantation rate were found between the different subgroups. The authors claimed that aforementioned algorithm is a powerful tool for embryo selection in TLS [40].

Milewski et al. create two predictive models for blastocyst development [41] and the transferred embryo implantation ability [42]. They evaluated the embryo morphokinetic parameters between embryos developed to blastocyst, and embryos did not reach blastocyst stage [41] as well as between implanted and non-implanted embryos [42]. Based on the findings and using statistical analysis, two models were generated which presented TLS as a good predictive instruments for embryo implantation but not as high as the model for blastocyst formation. Recently, Petersen et al. presented an appropriate algorithm for Day 3 of transferred embryos which is not dependent on culture conditions and fertilization method. The data was gathered retrospectively from a record of 3275 KID embryos transferred on Day 3 performed in 24 clinics. The new algorithm (KIDScore) was developed based on the six TLS parameters including one morphological and five morphokinetic events. Embryos were allocated to five categories, which predict the embryos' implantation potential. The algorithm was validated using a discrete data set of embryos cultured until Day 5 to examination of its ability to predict blastocyst formation. It is concluded that KIDScore could be considered as a "generally applicable Day-3 algorithm" which can be useful in "different clinical settings" [43]. Steadily, the effectiveness of the six embryo selection algorithms (ESAs) [15, 40, 44–47] was observed among 884 IVF or ICSI cycles. Validity of each ESA for detecting embryo implantation potential was determined using specificity, sensitivity, positive and negative predictive value (PPV and NPV), area under the receiver operating characteristic curve (AUC), and likelihood ratio (LR) regarding implantation rate in each model. Results showed the necessity of development in predictive algorithms according to the patients' characteristics, treatment protocols, and environmental factors. They believed that current ESAs may not work properly during application in other clinics [48]. Dominguez et al. combined TLS and proteomics to design a new model for the best embryo selection. They evaluated seven proteins in embryo culture media and find a correlation between them and embryo morphokinetics. The most relevant parameters were interleukin (IL-6) and cc2 among proteins and embryo time points, respectively. According to this relationship, an algorithm was considered for estimation embryo implantation rate. Embryos in the existence of IL-6 and 5–12 hours cc2 had remarkable implantation rate compared to other embryos [3].

Declared data showed that using embryo morphologic variables in combination with key time events leads to generate cumulative score models. It seems that these predictive algorithms integrate different variables and could not be easily adjusted to provide a globally accepted model. It is necessary to design in-house models which are specified for the same patients and conditions.

2.7. Different studies based on time-lapse observation

With the recent progress of TLS, a new opportunity is provided to study embryo developmental process accurately. TL monitoring offers a possibility to have exact observation on both early and late embryo morphokinetics and their correlation to embryo origin, fertilization methods, genetic abnormalities, and observer variability. In this section we review some of these studies.

To evaluate the influence of embryo origin by means of treatment-related factors on embryo morphokinetics, a cohort study was established among 1507 embryo from 243 patients. The results showed that blastocyst-stage embryos are more influenced by patients' characteristics than cleavage-stage embryos. Patients' age and dose of FSH have a positive correlation with delayed blastocyst development. It is also shown that embryos fertilized by ICSI have a significant faster first cleavage division than IVF originate embryos [49].

Minasi et al. examined that morphokinetic parameters of 928 blastocysts underwent preimplantation genetic screening (PGS). They reported no significant difference among euploid and aneuploid embryos regarding time-lapse morphokinetics and concluded that morphokinetic parameters can be used in combination with, not instead of, PGS for detecting embryo ploidy status [50]. Conversely, in a retrospective cohort study, a total of 460 embryos were cultured in TLS and biopsied on Day 3. Comparative genomic hybridization (CGH) microarray was performed for detecting aneuploidy. The result showed that some kinetic parameters including tPNF, t2, t5, cc2, and cc3 differ significantly among normal and aneuploid embryos [51].

Regarding the effect of intercellular communication on embryo development, a study was conducted on 765 good quality four-cell embryos. Four-cell embryos were investigated for intercellular contact point (ICCP) on Day 2 after insemination. The results showed that embryos with less than six ICCPs at the termination of four-cell stage have a decreased implantation potential when compared to those reaching six ICCPs by the end of four-cell stage (5 versus 38.5%). They concluded that discarding of embryos with poor morphology, abnormal cleavage, and fewer than six ICCPs at the four-cell stage results in a meaningful improvement in implantation rate [52].

To define the impact of fertilization methods on embryo morphokinetic, Bodri et al. evaluated 500 expanded blastocysts incubated in TLS retrospectively. The result indicated that IVF-fertilized embryos have a significant delay in early embryo developmental stages (pronucleus fading to t4) compared to embryos inseminated by ICSI, whereas IVF-fertilized embryos developed faster during blastocyst expansion stage. They reported a 1.5-hour time difference between standard IVF embryo and ICSI-fertilized embryo [53]. However, a definite conclusion needs further assessment with more studied cases.

For the first time, Sundvall et al. evaluate inter- and intra-observer inconsistency of time-lapse explanations. Three observers performed self-directed interpretations on time-lapse recordings on 158 fertilized embryos. Totally, the correlation was high for all of the examined parameters. Results showed close and strong interobserver agreement. The highest correlation was found for the timing of pronucleus breakdown, the completion of blastocyst hatching, and the appearance and disappearance of the first nucleus after the first division. There was also a perfect agreement for all cleavage stages. Two binary parameters including multinucleation and evenness of blastomeres at two-cell stage presented reasonable agreement. Intra-observer variability evaluation demonstrated comparable results for most parameters. The authors indicated that embryo morphokinetic factors can be used certainly for embryo viability prediction, even the recording interpret by a trainee operator [54].

2.8. Conclusion

Embryo selection criteria based on the current morphological evaluation do not associate with a high implantation or pregnancy rate. During the recent years, different studies based on a TLS have delivered new knowledge on embryo development proposing embryologists the chance to improve embryo evaluation and selection. Analysis of human embryo morphokinetics provides an improvement of implantation potential prediction at both early and late cleavage stages as well as prognosis potential to reach the blastocyst stage. Furthermore, TLS plays a key role in progress of SET policy to minimize multiple pregnancy and related complication. Moreover, embryo time-lapse monitoring reduces inter- or intra-observer variability. "Tele-embryology" may be considered as another advantage of TLS that allows monitoring embryos remotely via the Internet from any location. In addition TL monitoring collects large amount of data including recorded and stored images and videos which can be analyzed retrospectively. However, several studies presented positive outcomes and clinical validity of TLS; there are some limitations regarding this instrument. Some arguments remain regarding embryo exposure to light during image acquisition (every 5–15 min). It is a preference to plan guidelines on image capturing in terms of light wavelength, duration of lightening, and frequency of imaging. Likewise, there are restrictions in embryo rotation which make difficulties in the visual observation especially in the presence of cytoplasmic fragmentation or overlapping blastomeres. On the other hand, an important limitation in morphokinetic assessment is that the human embryo morphology is not a good figure of the chromosomal status. It is well known that embryos with good morphology may have aneuploidy, whereas suboptimal embryos may be euploid [21, 55]. Therefore, TLS should be applied in conjunction with PGS for detecting genetic abnormalities. Moreover, a number of confounding factors are recommended to effect timing of morphokinetic parameters including, oxygen tension, ovarian stimulation protocol, fertilization methods, type of culture media, smoking, and advanced age which should be considered in TLS researches.

Recently, some algorithms which are designed according to embryo morphokinetics suggested predicting embryo implantation and pregnancy potential. It states that the time points in these models are overlapped and the algorithms lose their predictive value when externally applied. Future properly designed study is needed to plan a common classification for key time points and time intervals that are accepted worldwide.

In conclusion, implantation rate should be considered as the first outcome and take-home baby rate as the final outcome to evaluating success of this new technology. Some researchers believed that embryo selection via TLS should remain an experimental policy due to lack of evidence-based medicine to sufficiently assess the safety and effectiveness of this equipment. However, it is important to know that TLS is a powerful noninvasive technology for the study of embryo development which offers a wide-range document of morphological and dynamic parameters about each embryo. The system should be evaluated for cost/benefit ratio effectiveness in individual laboratory.

Author details

Nasim Tabibnejad

Address all correspondence to: nasimtabibnejad@ssu.ac.ir

Research and Clinical Infertility Center, Yazd Reproductive Sciences Institute, Shahid Sadoughi University of Medical Sciences, Yazd, Iran

References

[1] Wong CC, Loewke KE, Bossert NL, Behr B, De Jonge CJ, Baer TM, et al. Non-invasive imaging of human embryos before embryonic genome activation predicts development to the blastocyst stage. Nature Biotechnology. 2010;**28**(10):1115-1121

[2] Meseguer M, Rubio I, Cruz M, Basile N, Marcos J, Requena A. Embryo incubation and selection in a time-lapse monitoring system improves pregnancy outcome compared with a standard incubator: A retrospective cohort study. Fertility and Sterility. 2012;**98**(6):1481-1489 e10

[3] Dominguez F, Meseguer M, Aparicio-Ruiz B, Piqueras P, Quinonero A, Simon C. New strategy for diagnosing embryo implantation potential by combining proteomics and time-lapse technologies. Fertility and Sterility. 2015;**104**(4):908-914

[4] Adamson GD, Abusief ME, Palao L, Witmer J, Palao LM, Gvakharia M. Improved implantation rates of day 3 embryo transfers with the use of an automated time-lapse-enabled test to aid in embryo selection. Fertility and Sterility. 2016;**105**(2):369-375 e6

[5] Kirkegaard K, Kesmodel US, Hindkjaer JJ, Ingerslev HJ. Time-lapse parameters as predictors of blastocyst development and pregnancy outcome in embryos from good prognosis patients: A prospective cohort study. Human Reproduction. 2013;**28**(10):2643-2651

[6] Milewski R, Czerniecki J, Kuczynska A, Stankiewicz B, Kuczynski W. Morphokinetic parameters as a source of information concerning embryo developmental and implantation potential. Ginekologia Polska. 2016;**87**(10):677-684

[7] Rubio I, Galan A, Larreategui Z, Ayerdi F, Bellver J, Herrero J, et al. Clinical validation of embryo culture and selection by morphokinetic analysis: A randomized, controlled trial of the EmbryoScope. Fertility and Sterility. 2014;**102**(5):1287-1294, e5

[8] Desai N, Ploskonka S, Goodman LR, Austin C, Goldberg J, Falcone T. Analysis of embryo morphokinetics, multinucleation and cleavage anomalies using continuous time-lapse monitoring in blastocyst transfer cycles. Reproductive Biology and Endocrinology: RB&E. 2014;**12**:54

[9] Conaghan J, Chen AA, Willman SP, Ivani K, Chenette PE, Boostanfar R, et al. Improving embryo selection using a computer-automated time-lapse image analysis test plus day 3 morphology: Results from a prospective multicenter trial. Fertility and Sterility. 2013;**100**(2):412-419 e5

[10] Diamond MP, Suraj V, Behnke EJ, Yang X, Angle MJ, Lambe-Steinmiller JC, et al. Using the Eeva Test adjunctively to traditional day 3 morphology is informative for consistent embryo assessment within a panel of embryologists with diverse experience. Journal of Assisted Reproduction and Genetics. 2015;**32**(1):61-68

[11] Herrero J, Tejera A, Albert C, Vidal C, de los Santos MJ, Meseguer M. A time to look back: Analysis of morphokinetic characteristics of human embryo development. Fertility and Sterility. 2013;**100**(6):1602-1609, e1-e4

[12] Motato Y, de los Santos MJ, Escriba MJ, Ruiz BA, Remohi J, Meseguer M. Morphokinetic analysis and embryonic prediction for blastocyst formation through an integrated time-lapse system. Fertility and Sterility. 2016;**105**(2):376-384, e9

[13] Park H, Bergh C, Selleskog U, Thurin-Kjellberg A, Lundin K. No benefit of culturing embryos in a closed system compared with a conventional incubator in terms of number of good quality embryos: Results from an RCT. Human Reproduction. 2015;**30**(2):268-275

[14] Nakahara T, Iwase A, Goto M, Harata T, Suzuki M, Ienaga M, et al. Evaluation of the safety of time-lapse observations for human embryos. Journal of Assisted Reproduction and Genetics. 2010;**27**(2-3):93-96

[15] Cruz M, Garrido N, Herrero J, Perez-Cano I, Munoz M, Meseguer M. Timing of cell division in human cleavage-stage embryos is linked with blastocyst formation and quality. Reproductive Biomedicine Online. 2012;**25**(4):371-381

[16] Kirkegaard K, Hindkjaer JJ, Grondahl ML, Kesmodel US, Ingerslev HJ. A randomized clinical trial comparing embryo culture in a conventional incubator with a time-lapse incubator. Journal of Assisted Reproduction and Genetics. 2012;**29**(6):565-572

[17] Wu YG, Lazzaroni-Tealdi E, Wang Q, Zhang L, Barad DH, Kushnir VA, et al. Different effectiveness of closed embryo culture system with time-lapse imaging (EmbryoScope(TM)) in comparison to standard manual embryology in good and poor prognosis patients: A prospectively randomized pilot study. Reproductive Biology and Endocrinology: RB&E. 2016;**14**(1):49

[18] Goodman LR, Goldberg J, Falcone T, Austin C, Desai N. Does the addition of time-lapse morphokinetics in the selection of embryos for transfer improve pregnancy rates? A randomized controlled trial. Fertility and Sterility. 2016;**105**(2):275-285, e10

[19] Alomar M, Tasiaux H, Remacle S, George F, Paul D, Donnay I. Kinetics of fertilization and development, and sex ratio of bovine embryos produced using the semen of different bulls. Animal Reproduction Science. 2008;**107**(1-2):48-61

[20] Bermejo-Alvarez P, Roberts RM, Rosenfeld CS. Effect of glucose concentration during in vitro culture of mouse embryos on development to blastocyst, success of embryo transfer, and litter sex ratio. Molecular Reproduction and Development. 2012;**79**(5):329-336

[21] Alfarawati S, Fragouli E, Colls P, Stevens J, Gutierrez-Mateo C, Schoolcraft WB, et al. The relationship between blastocyst morphology, chromosomal abnormality, and embryo gender. Fertility and Sterility. 2011;**95**(2):520-524

[22] Hentemann MA, Briskemyr S, Bertheussen K. Blastocyst transfer and gender: IVF versus ICSI. Journal of Assisted Reproduction and Genetics. 2009;**26**(8):433-436

[23] Serdarogullari M, Findikli N, Goktas C, Sahin O, Ulug U, Yagmur E, et al. Comparison of gender-specific human embryo development characteristics by time-lapse technology. Reproductive Biomedicine Online. 2014;**29**(2):193-199

[24] Weston G, Osianlis T, Catt J, Vollenhoven B. Blastocyst transfer does not cause a sex-ratio imbalance. Fertility and Sterility. 2009;**92**(4):1302-1305

[25] Bodri D, Kawachiya S, Sugimoto T, Yao Serna J, Kato R, Matsumoto T. Time-lapse variables and embryo gender: A retrospective analysis of 81 live births obtained following minimal stimulation and single embryo transfer. Journal of Assisted Reproduction and Genetics. 2016;**33**(5):589-596

[26] Bronet F, Nogales MC, Martinez E, Ariza M, Rubio C, Garcia-Velasco JA, et al. Is there a relationship between time-lapse parameters and embryo sex? Fertility and Sterility. 2015;**103**(2):396-401 e2

[27] Chavez SL, Loewke KE, Han J, Moussavi F, Colls P, Munne S, et al. Dynamic blastomere behaviour reflects human embryo ploidy by the four-cell stage. Nature Communications. 2012;**3**:1251

[28] Stensen MH, Tanbo TG, Storeng R, Abyholm T, Fedorcsak P. Fragmentation of human cleavage-stage embryos is related to the progression through meiotic and mitotic cell cycles. Fertility and Sterility. 2015;**103**(2):374-381, e4

[29] Requena A, Cruz M, Agudo D, Pacheco A, Garcia-Velasco JA. Type of gonadotropin during controlled ovarian stimulation affects the endocrine profile in follicular fluid and apoptosis rate in cumulus cells. European Journal of Obstetrics, Gynecology, and Reproductive Biology. 2016;**197**:142-146

[30] Munoz M, Cruz M, Humaidan P, Garrido N, Perez-Cano I, Meseguer M. The type of GnRH analogue used during controlled ovarian stimulation influences early embryo developmental kinetics: A time-lapse study. European Journal of Obstetrics, Gynecology, and Reproductive Biology. 2013;**168**(2):167-172

[31] Gurbuz AS, Gode F, Uzman MS, Ince B, Kaya M, Ozcimen N, et al. GnRH agonist triggering affects the kinetics of embryo development: A comparative study. Journal of Ovarian Research. 2016;**9**:22

[32] Munoz M, Cruz M, Humaidan P, Garrido N, Perez-Cano I, Meseguer M. Dose of recombinant FSH and oestradiol concentration on day of HCG affect embryo development kinetics. Reproductive Biomedicine Online. 2012;**25**(4):382-389

[33] Morbeck DE, Krisher RL, Herrick JR, Baumann NA, Matern D, Moyer T. Composition of commercial media used for human embryo culture. Fertility and Sterility. 2014;**102**(3):759-766 e9

[34] Basile N, Morbeck D, Garcia-Velasco J, Bronet F, Meseguer M. Type of culture media does not affect embryo kinetics: A time-lapse analysis of sibling oocytes. Human Reproduction. 2013;**28**(3):634-641

[35] Hardarson T, Bungum M, Conaghan J, Meintjes M, Chantilis SJ, Molnar L, et al. Noninferiority, randomized, controlled trial comparing embryo development using media developed for sequential or undisturbed culture in a time-lapse setup. Fertility and Sterility. 2015;**104**(6):1452-1459 e1-e4

[36] Costa-Borges N, Belles M, Meseguer M, Galliano D, Ballesteros A, Calderon G. Blastocyst development in single medium with or without renewal on day 3: A prospective

cohort study on sibling donor oocytes in a time-lapse incubator. Fertility and Sterility. 2016;**105**(3):707-713

[37] Meseguer M, Herrero J, Tejera A, Hilligsoe KM, Ramsing NB, Remohi J. The use of morphokinetics as a predictor of embryo implantation. Human Reproduction. 2011;**26**(10): 2658-2671

[38] Freour T, Le Fleuter N, Lammers J, Splingart C, Reignier A, Barriere P. External validation of a time-lapse prediction model. Fertility and Sterility. 2015;**103**(4):917-922

[39] Liu Y, Chapple V, Feenan K, Roberts P, Matson P. Time-lapse deselection model for human day 3 in vitro fertilization embryos: The combination of qualitative and quantitative measures of embryo growth. Fertility and Sterility. 2016;**105**(3):656-662 e1

[40] Basile N, Vime P, Florensa M, Aparicio Ruiz B, Garcia Velasco JA, Remohi J, et al. The use of morphokinetics as a predictor of implantation: A multicentric study to define and validate an algorithm for embryo selection. Human Reproduction. 2015;**30**(2):276-283

[41] Milewski R, Kuc P, Kuczynska A, Stankiewicz B, Lukaszuk K, Kuczynski W. A predictive model for blastocyst formation based on morphokinetic parameters in time-lapse monitoring of embryo development. Journal of Assisted Reproduction and Genetics. 2015;**32**(4):571-579

[42] Milewski R, Milewska AJ, Kuczynska A, Stankiewicz B, Kuczynski W. Do morphokinetic data sets inform pregnancy potential? Journal of Assisted Reproduction and Genetics. 2016;**33**(3):357-365

[43] Petersen BM, Boel M, Montag M, Gardner DK. Development of a generally applicable morphokinetic algorithm capable of predicting the implantation potential of embryos transferred on Day 3. Human Reproduction. 2016;**31**(10):2231-2244

[44] Azzarello A, Hoest T, Mikkelsen AL. The impact of pronuclei morphology and dynamicity on live birth outcome after time-lapse culture. Human Reproduction. 2012;**27**(9): 2649-2657

[45] Campbell A, Fishel S, Bowman N, Duffy S, Sedler M, Hickman CF. Modelling a risk classification of aneuploidy in human embryos using non-invasive morphokinetics. Reproductive Biomedicine Online. 2013;**26**(5):477-485

[46] Chamayou S, Patrizio P, Storaci G, Tomaselli V, Alecci C, Ragolia C, et al. The use of morphokinetic parameters to select all embryos with full capacity to implant. Journal of Assisted Reproduction and Genetics. 2013;**30**(5):703-710

[47] Dal Canto M, Coticchio G, Mignini Renzini M, De Ponti E, Novara PV, Brambillasca F, et al. Cleavage kinetics analysis of human embryos predicts development to blastocyst and implantation. Reproductive Biomedicine Online. 2012;**25**(5):474-480

[48] Barrie A, Homburg R, McDowell G, Brown J, Kingsland C, Troup S. Examining the efficacy of six published time-lapse imaging embryo selection algorithms to predict implantation to demonstrate the need for the development of specific, in-house morphokinetic selection algorithms. Fertility and Sterility. 2017; 107(3):613-621

[49] Kirkegaard K, Sundvall L, Erlandsen M, Hindkjaer JJ, Knudsen UB, Ingerslev HJ. Timing of human preimplantation embryonic development is confounded by embryo origin. Human Reproduction. 2016;**31**(2):324-331

[50] Minasi MG, Colasante A, Riccio T, Ruberti A, Casciani V, Scarselli F, et al. Correlation between aneuploidy, standard morphology evaluation and morphokinetic development in 1730 biopsied blastocysts: A consecutive case series study. Human Reproduction. 2016;**31**(10):2245-2254

[51] Chawla M, Fakih M, Shunnar A, Bayram A, Hellani A, Perumal V, et al. Morphokinetic analysis of cleavage stage embryos and its relationship to aneuploidy in a retrospective time-lapse imaging study. Journal of Assisted Reproduction and Genetics. 2015;**32**(1):69-75

[52] Liu Y, Chapple V, Feenan K, Roberts P, Matson P. Clinical significance of intercellular contact at the four-cell stage of human embryos, and the use of abnormal cleavage patterns to identify embryos with low implantation potential: A time-lapse study. Fertility and Sterility. 2015;**103**(6):1485-1491 e1

[53] Bodri D, Sugimoto T, Serna JY, Kondo M, Kato R, Kawachiya S, et al. Influence of different oocyte insemination techniques on early and late morphokinetic parameters: Retrospective analysis of 500 time-lapse monitored blastocysts. Fertility and Sterility. 2015;**104**(5):1175-1181 e1-e2

[54] Sundvall L, Ingerslev HJ, Breth Knudsen U, Kirkegaard K. Inter- and intra-observer variability of time-lapse annotations. Human Reproduction. 2013;**28**(12):3215-3221

[55] Ziebe S, Lundin K, Loft A, Bergh C, Nyboe Andersen A, Selleskog U, et al. FISH analysis for chromosomes 13, 16, 18, 21, 22, X and Y in all blastomeres of IVF pre-embryos from 144 randomly selected donated human oocytes and impact on pre-embryo morphology. Human Reproduction. 2003;**18**(12):2575-2581

Chapter 4

Methods for Spatio-Temporal Analysis of Embryo Cleavage In Vitro

Anna Leida Mölder,
Juan Carlos Fierro-González and Aisha Khan

Additional information is available at the end of the chapter

http://dx.doi.org/10.5772/intechopen.69650

Abstract

Automated or semiautomated time-lapse analysis of early stage embryo images during the cleavage stage can give insight into the timing of mitosis, regularity of both division timing and pattern, as well as cell lineage. Simultaneous monitoring of molecular processes enables the study of connections between genetic expression and cell physiology and development. The study of live embryos poses not only new requirements on the hardware and embryo-holding equipment but also indirectly on analytical software and data analysis as four-dimensional video sequencing of embryos easily creates high quantities of data. The ability to continuously film and automatically analyze growing embryos gives new insights into temporal embryo development by studying morphokinetics as well as morphology. Until recently, this was not possible unless by a tedious manual process. In recent years, several methods have been developed that enable this dynamic monitoring of live embryos. Here we describe three methods with variations in hardware and software analysis and give examples of the outcomes. Together, these methods open a window to new information in developmental embryology, as embryo division pattern and lineage are studied in vivo.

Keywords: embryo cleavage, time-lapse analysis, morphokinetics, embryo profiling, phylogenetics, cell lineage

1. Introduction

Despite 30 years of practice, the success rate for implantation of embryos into the uterus in in vitro fertilization (IVF) is still only around 30% [1, 2]. Consequently, when transferring embryos from in vitro culture and implanting them, it is critical that only the best embryos are selected. This will not only optimize the chance of live birth but also reduce the need for multiple embryo transfer, with the subsequent risk of twin pregnancy and the neonatal complications and associated maternal pregnancy-related health problems. Though cultivation methods have improved, embryo selection is still largely based on manual evaluation of morphological criteria, and much research has been done in identifying morphological features correlated with embryo health. Other methods such as genetic screening and metabolic profiles of culture media exist, but have not yet proven to increase pregnancy rates [3–9]. There is an ongoing discussion concerning the relevance of embryo morphology in quality assessment [10], but it is likely that it will continue to play a large part in IVF embryo evaluation also in the future. Traditionally, embryo quality assessment has been performed by manual inspection using light microscopy at intermittent time points during embryo development. Novel technical solutions have recently made it possible to monitor embryos continuously using time-lapse imaging, opening new possibilities for embryo evaluation based on dynamic properties.

It has been shown that the timing of key occurrences within the embryo can vary greatly between embryos that have similar morphological appearance at the end of the recording period and that embryo morphology can change in a matter of hours [11–14], emphasizing the fact that dynamic monitoring is preferred over intermittent monitoring of embryos. An important endpoint for embryo studies is the timing of embryo cleavage, which has been shown to correlate to embryo viability and implantation potential [15–18]. For research purposes, tracking of cell lineage and cell positioning within the early embryo provides important information to understand pluripotency. Embryos are also a good model for the study of developmental biology and three-dimensional cellular interaction. The ability to continuously film and analyze growing embryos gives new insights into temporal embryo development by studying morphokinetics as well as morphology. Until recently, this was only possible by a tedious manual process. Although currently some human IVF laboratories have started to use time-lapse technology to monitor embryo cleavage and growth, further description of the technology and its potential is needed. The focus of this chapter is on the methods used to study living early embryos over time and the possibilities they render as new tools for embryological research and clinical application.

2. The role of live imaging in embryology

Conventional microscopy suffers from several drawbacks, such as requiring sample fixing and only providing static information in an intermittent manner. The complete understanding of cell division and development requires a dynamic perspective on an individual cell level as most information on cell response to environment, dynamic gene expression and timing would be missed in a static analysis. In recent years, the imaging technologies have provided new tools in microscopy, sample handling, and hardware and software for live imaging of individual cells. There are several examples of single cell [19–22] and single molecule monitoring in living cells, using both marker-based and marker-free approaches.

Fluorescent tags enable the tracing of specific proteins and measurement of their characteristics to study gene expression, protein localization, and function and protein-protein interaction. By using several markers simultaneously, it is possible to track several proteins or gene expressions at once. With time-lapse microscopy, intracellular events can be linked to external factors such as cell-cell interaction and ultimate cell fate. These methods give us remarkable new insights into the dynamics of gene expression, cellular interactions, and heterogeneous processes. In fluorescence imaging, a laser is used to excite the fluorophores at a particular wavelength. Full field epifluorescence can then be used to measure the light as the fluorescent tags emit light while returning to their unexcited molecular state [23]. In confocal imaging, a pinhole in combination with focused laser light is introduced to effectively reduce background fluorescence and allows optical sectioning of the sample by mechanical scanning. Varying the pinhole will effectively vary the thickness of the sample being imaged, the image resolution, and the acquisition time.

For some applications, the use of fluorescent tags is not feasible. By continuously filming embryo material some important information on cell outline, position, shape, and texture can be extracted from the time-lapse sequences without the use of fluorescent markers. By matching and tracking, this information can be combined to a timing profile of the dividing embryo, detecting temporal location of division and tracking cell lineage over time. Using computer vision in combination with a noninvasive imaging method makes it possible to continuously study embryo growth with minimal sample interference. Fluorescence imaging allows the noninvasive measurement of gene expression and intracellular characteristics, while marker-free light microscopy allows the tracking of cellular size, shape, and behavior over time in response to molecular changes. This combination gives us the possibility to directly monitor cellular responses and changes in gene expression in response to the environment. The result is a cellular model that can bridge the molecular scale to the cellular, mapping the actual connections between the chemical and the biological world.

3. Noninvasive techniques for embryo imaging

Currently, a set of biotechniques has been successfully applied to mouse and human embryo imaging. This technique includes the addition of a fluorescent marker and marker-free methods. For research purposes, the addition of fluorescent proteins can be considered a noninvasive method, if the protocol used does not significantly disturb embryo growth. For clinical applications in human embryology, no markers of any kind can be used. In this section, we will refer to fluorescent marker methods as noninvasive, and specify the "truly" noninvasive method as "marker free."

3.1. Fluorescence imaging

Adding fluorescent proteins (FP) is a standard way to selectively study specific intracellular targets [24]. The most common fluorescent tag is the green fluorescent protein (GFP) [25], derived from the jellyfish *Aequorea Victoria* [26]. The FP is introduced by transfection or microinjection of a plasmid DNA expressing vector, carrying the genetic code for the protein. By tagging a biologically functional protein of interest with the FP, a specific pathway can be tracked. The use of FPs enables a straightforward way to locate the protein within the cell, but this can have drawbacks. Phototoxicity may occur at short enough wavelengths and at high laser excitation intensities [27]. Also, a transient expression of FP may result in higher-than-normal levels of the functional protein accompanying it, which may have unforeseen effects on the dynamic behavior of the entire system. Alternatively, the FP can be integrated into the genome using targeted genome editing technologies like CRISPR-Cas9 (M3), in which case the number of plasmid copies per cell will no longer affect the protein concentration. Control experiments are necessary to establish the effect of the FP study method, which may differ for each host system or experimental environment.

FP can also be used to study the dynamics around the FP binding site by fluorescence recovery after photobleaching (FRAP) [28]. In FRAP, a fluorophore is covalently attached to the molecule of interest. The fluorophore is intentionally photobleached using incident laser light. The diffusion of the molecules can now be quantified by studying the gradual brightening of the photobleached spot, as fresh fluorophores migrate into this area. Three closely related techniques are the fluorescence loss in photobleaching (FLIP), fluorescence decay after photoactivation (FDAP), and fluorescence correlation spectroscopy (FCS) [29]. Fluorescence resonance energy transfer (FRET) (sometimes also called Förster resonance energy transfer) can be used to study protein-protein interactions [30]. In this case, a donor fluorophore is placed in an excited state by incident laser light, and the energy held in the excited molecular state is transferred to an acceptor fluorophore which must be in close proximity (typically less than ten nanometers). When two molecules under study are labelled with the donor and acceptor fluorophores, respectively, the detected light from the acceptor fluorophore indicates that the two molecules are in close proximity.

A number of studies have used fluorescent markers using various imaging modalities to study protein movement within the embryo [31–34] and using embryonic stem cells [35, 36].

3.2. Marker-free microscopy

Currently, IVF centers or clinics are using two main techniques for embryo imaging: Hoffman modulation contrast imaging (HMC) (sometimes referred to as white light) [37, 38] and dark-field imaging (DF) [39]. For research purposes, CARS [40] and light sheet microscopy [41] are also becoming increasingly common. HMC was standard before time-lapse imaging of IVF embryos came in use and is still used in manual microscopy set ups. Consequently, images from time-lapse sequencing resemble the microscopy images to which embryologists are accustomed, an advantage when annotating images and comparing manual and computational approaches. HMC is best suited for imaging internal cell detail. On the other hand, Darkfield gives better detail to edge structures such as cell membranes, and more accurately to detect and track cell outlines.

Darkfield imaging is an imaging method that excludes any unscattered light, causing the samples to appear brighter on a darker background and enhancing the contrast of the imaged and unstained sample [42]. It is a simple yet effective method to noninvasively enhance sample contrast but has the disadvantage of low light levels available for collection. To compensate, the sample must be strongly illuminated and the heavy light exposure can cause sample damage. However, the low light level also means the image is almost entirely free from optical artifacts. Darkfield microscopy is most useful for studying boundary structures with a high difference in refractive index and imaging cell membranes is, for instance, more effective than internal cell structures. It is best suited for thin samples with high differences in refractive index (such as for sharp edges) and for thick samples, artifacts may occur.

HMC Imaging was invented by Hoffman in 1975 [43]. Today, it is a common technique for noninvasive contrast enhancement of biological samples. Its advantages include good contrast, low light exposure, excellent resolution, and a short depth of field, with the opportunity of focal sectioning at a resolution controllable by the numerical aperture of the objective. The ability to section is also influenced by the sample homogeneity. The disadvantages include strong optical artifacts and image appearance unsuitable for computerized image processing. HMC is commonly been used for embryology studies and has been included in a number of commercial products.

4. Challenges in live embryo imaging

Although advances have been achieved in techniques for live single-cell imaging in recent years, several challenges still exist for wider implementation. An experimental design for long-term imaging and analysis must ensure not only high-quality imaging but also long-term support for sample vitality and appropriate computational methods for the analysis. Observing embryo in vitro requires an incubator environment to provide optimal living conditions or the sample during the imaging period. Temperature changes can affect the function of physiological processes as well as reaction kinetics and the challenge will increase with the length of the study sequence. One solution is the installation of an incubation flow chamber on the microscope, reducing the amount of gas and liquid to sustain the sample to a small volume, but suffering from drawbacks such as the risk of introducing condensation on the incubator chamber surfaces. Another approach is to integrate the microscopy optics in an incubator chamber, posing demands on the microscope optics and electronics to function in a humid, temperate atmosphere. A limited number of commercial solutions exist, which combine incubation capabilities with imaging hardware. With any of these solutions, the embryo medium and container must not introduce imaging artifacts such as light reflecting surfaces, auto-fluorescence, or excessive medium volumes in the light path. Another challenge is the loading and retrieval of cells from the mounting chamber, a process that may cause loss of cell identification. For IVF, several combinations of incubators and microscopes exists [44], either as integrated solutions or in the form of a microscope designed for use inside an incubator. So far, no difference has yet been seen in growth and implantation rates of embryos grown in the standard intermittent incubator system and a time-lapse incubator system [45–47]. One study found a higher rate of miscarriage for the time-lapse group, indicating there are reasons for caution. However, the same study noted no effect on pregnancy rates or embryo health prior to implantation [48].

In nonhuman IVF, phase contrast microscopy is commonly utilized instead of HMC. Phase contrast microscopy is similar to HMC in that it gives high level of image detail at the expense of image artifacts in the form of halos around sample objects. The varying appearance of embryos of different species will affect the decision of which optical system to use. Some species have dark, dense-appearing embryos (e.g., pig), while others are more translucent (e.g., mouse). As a consequence the optimal optical system for a given embryo species vary, and any appropriate analytical software must be chosen accordingly. Single-cell studies using darkfield imaging is limited by the hardware to the 4–6 cell stage. Using focal sectioning in HMC, it is possible to image the entire embryo from zygote to blastocyst stage, but any automated analysis becomes increasingly difficult with increasing cell number as the out-of-focus image details cannot be removed, despite the sectioning. In humans, the compaction at the 9–16-cell stage involves a reduction in visibility of cell boundaries and may represent a feasible stage for automated detection beyond the 8-cell stage. The cavitation and blastocyst formation stages also offer opportunities for automated analysis of images, covering expansion and collapse events.

In fluorescence time-lapse imaging of nonhuman mammalian embryos, the life time of the fluorophores is limited, an effect referred to as *photobleaching* [27]. Bleaching can be limited by reducing exposure, but ultimately sets a limit to the duration of the imaging sequence. The most severe cause of concern is the toxic effects caused by the exposure to intense laser light for a prolonged period of time. This *phototoxicity* can be limited by minimizing laser exposure using mechanical fast shutters or switching LEDs, but any shutters will quickly reach the end of their life span in a continuous time-lapse imaging set up. Switching at 1 Hz, a shutter will open and close a million times in about 12 days. In all cases, an efficient microscopy control software is necessary.

There is a trade-off between information gathered and potentially harmful sample exposure, and the frequency of image capture must be carefully chosen depending on the study end-point and the expected frequency of the dynamics under study. In the case of simultaneous monitoring of multiple samples, two solutions exist. In *scanning*, either the imaging hardware or sample is moved and repositioned at each image capture. In this case there is a trade-off (limited by the moving mechanics) between samples imaged and images captured per sample. In *full-field,* the image captured includes all samples simultaneously. In this case, there is instead a trade-off between the number of samples imaged and the image resolution available to each sample.

For two-dimensional imaging, full-field techniques are the most efficient as they capture the entire field of view in one single exposure. However, the stability of the system becomes critical as the time-lapse sequence length increases. *Focal drift* remains a problem and an autofocus mechanism or a method for user input to correct may be needed.

Even with moderate capture frequency, the amount of data from time-lapse studies can quickly build up to terabytes or more, especially if data is recorded simultaneously in multiple dimensions and imaging modalities. Consequently, both *data storage*, efficient *access to data* for analysis and the *post-acquisition analysis* itself must be considered. A small amount of video data may be analyzed manually, but this method quickly becomes cumbersome and time-consuming and automatic or semiautomatic methods are necessary. Manual evaluation of images is also prone to errors and inter-observer variability [49, 50]. It is often beneficial if the intended analysis can be considered already at the image capture stage so that acquisition, image quality, and hardware set up can be optimized upfront. Several open source software applications exist for the analysis of video sequences. Unfortunately, they are generally not suited for more advanced analysis of multidimensional data, which is often the case in embryo studies, where three-dimensional scanning or focal sectioning is used to capture data in multiple dimensions. Specialized solutions tailored to the data are also often both faster and more accurate than a general purpose application. The development of analytical tools hinges on access to *verification data*, for example, in the form of annotated image data for ground truth. With the increasing amount of generated image data, the availability of such training data has become a significant bottleneck. The solution, increased sharing and open access to data and annotations, requires standardized methods for data management, format, and metadata storage. To this end, open-source bioimage database systems such as OMERO [51] are an important step.

The optimal *choice of analysis* differs widely with the experimental set up and the aim of the study. Often, an initial analytical step is the identification of cell outlines in images. There are several ways to detect and track cell outlines in embryo imaging, both segmentation-based (requiring an identification of embryonic cell outlines), segmentation-free [52–55], or a combination of these [56]. Usually, a correctly performed segmentation [54, 57–59] provides the most detailed information on cell position, shape, and outline, but is computationally also the more challenging.

No single set of experimental conditions for long-term imaging can be used universally. Each biological question and model requires its own specific combination of hardware and software tools and must often be customized. Solutions to these challenges will enable important discoveries in embryology in the future. Kang et al. [60] and Turksen [61] provide useful summaries of protocols for fluorescent labelling and the imaging and tracking of stem cell, respectively. The following three sections exemplify successful time-lapse imaging methodologies for both human and nonhuman embryos with solutions to the experimental challenges using three very different approaches.

5. Method 1: three-dimensional mouse embryo morphology using fluorescent markers

To understand compaction, cell lineage, cell rearrangement and dynamic behavior of embryonic cells during the cleavage phase, and dynamic imaging is necessary. This project studied the role of filopodia formation in compaction, apical constriction, pluripotent cell internalization, and cell positioning prior to embryo compaction, which is believed to be important for pluripotent development of embryonic cells. In addition, intracellular processes are monitored using a variety of targeted fluorescently tagged proteins and transcription factors.

With fluorescence microscopy, we can selectively excite and visualize fluorescent proteins as a marker in living tissue. The discovery of genetically encoded fluorescent proteins (FPs) permits the quantitative analysis of most cellular proteins including monitoring of their distribution and dynamics [62]. Fluorescence imaging is a technique that perfectly addresses problems in embryonic development, because of the need to study embryos in vivo. In confocal microscopy, in contrast to widefield fluorescence imaging, the detector pinhole blocks fluorescence from areas that lie out of focus [63]. This allows confocal imaging to reduce some of the scattering effects elicited by widefield fluorescence microscopy. However, scanning a single section implies the excitation and, therefore, damaging off-focus areas above and below the focal plane. In addition, the pinhole will also exclude scattered signal photons emitted from the focal plane as they travel away from the specimen. Therefore, widefield and confocal imaging are methods best suited for thin samples of less than ~40 μm. To study the events occurring deeper in the mouse embryo, which is about 100 μm in diameter (70 m of cellular portion plus the zona pellucida), requires the use of two-photon excitation fluorescence microscopy.

Two-photon excitation (2PE) fluorescence microscopy is a way to limit phototoxicity in the sample and to extend the imaging time and depth at high resolution and contrast [64]. In 2PE, two photons of half the excitation energy are needed to place the FP in the excited state. A focused laser is used in 2PE to generate higher intensity localized in the area of the focal plane, which results in excitation limited to a very small focal volume (typically of ~0.1 μm^3). A combination of confocal and two-photon excitation (2PE) fluorescence microscopy can be used to follow and characterize different morphogenetic changes in developing embryos such as cell division, polarity, filopodia formation and dynamics, compaction, and blastocyst cavitation (**Figure 1**). For this aim, specific fluorescently tagged proteins or peptides are used to label nuclear, cytoplasmic, or membrane constituents and optimized confocal and 2PE fluorescence imaging methods [29, 31, 65]. These imaging conditions allow the scan of a single embryo at intervals down to less than 60 s and reconstruction of 3D embryo morphology using Imaris (Bitplane AG) or ZEN (Zeiss) software. For long-term imaging sessions positioning software (Zeiss Zen) is used to image 20–30 embryos cultured next to each other (**Figure 1**). Thanks to the high-sensitive detectors of confocal and 2PE fluorescence microscopes, it is possible to perform long-term imaging sessions lasting more than 24 h, without this affecting the health and integrity of the mouse embryos. Thus it is possible to follow in an overnight imaging session cell dynamics in 20–30 embryos. Images are captured at intervals of 40 min from eight-cell stage to blastocyst (an interval of about 36 h). Capturing fluorescent imaging together with brightfield optics makes it possible to monitor simultaneously cell and molecular dynamics (**Figure 1D**).

For the simultaneous subcellular study of proteins at different stages of development, it is possible to study the dynamics of subcellular markers from zygote to blastocyst stage. For this purpose, DNA constructs in the pCS2+ expression vector [66] and synthesized capped RNA (using the Ambion mMessage mMachine SP6 transcription kit) are used. Capped marker-GFP RNA is injected into one-cell stage embryos. For nulcei, H2B-RFP is commonly used as marker, whereas memb-mCherry, Ecad-RFP, Ecad-GFP, or Ezrin-RFP can be used for membrane monitoring (**Figure 1**) [32, 34, 65]. **Figure 1C** shows an example of using the nuclear marker H2B-GFP and the membrane marker Ecad-GFP. Polarity events can be studied using Ezrin-GFP. Ezrin is expressed homogeneously in all cells before it becomes polarized during embryonic compaction [67] (**Figure 1B**). Hence, colocalization with Ezrin-GFP is an excellent way to study the dynamics and distribution of any protein of interest during compaction and cell polarity.

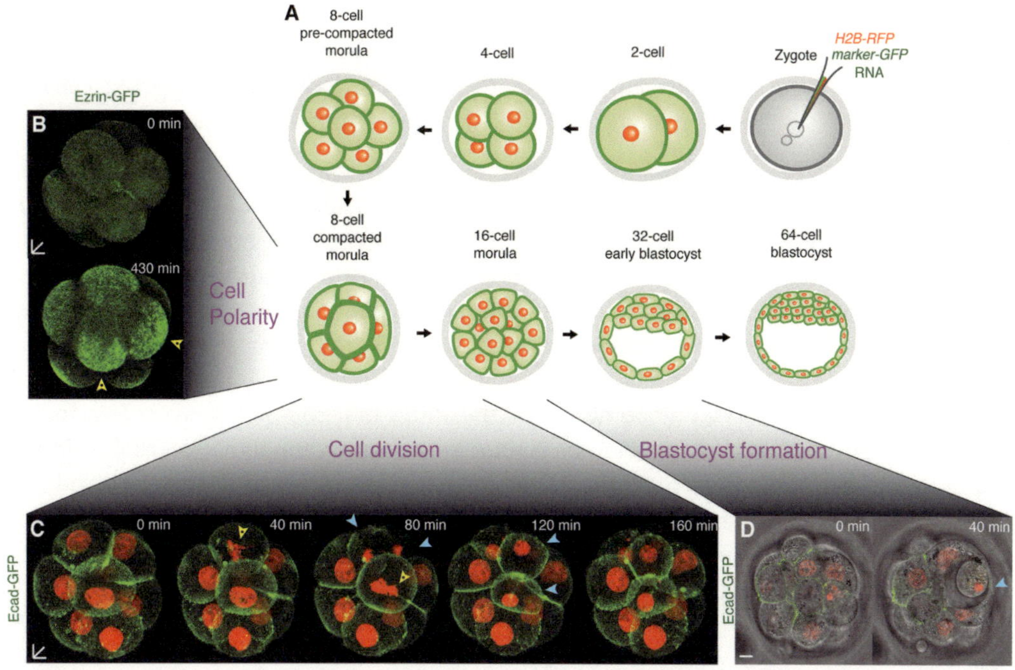

Figure 1. (A) Injection of nuclear (H2B-RFP) and cytoplasmic or membrane markers (marker-GFP) RNA at one cell stage, showing morphogenetic changes during mouse embryo development. (B) Cell polarity events (arrowheads) are observed at eight-cell stage visualized with the protein Ezrin-GFP. (C) Monitoring cytokinesis and timing of cell division using the membrane marker Ecad-GFP and nuclear marker H2B-RFP; Chromatin condensation is highlighted by dotted arrowheads, and cell division by plain arrowheads. (D) Cavitation (arrowhead) during blastocyst formation is observed with bright field optics combined with fluorescence imaging of membrane and nuclear markers (Ecad-GFP and H2B-RFP). Scale bar, 10 μm.

6. Method 2: cell lineage studies of human embryos using machine learning

This method focuses on automated monitoring of human embryonic cells in dark field time-lapse microscopy images of embryos with the goal to develop methods to segment, detect, localize the embryonic cells at each time step, and perform cell lineage analysis on a complete sequence. The result is a helpful tool for embryologists and IVF clinicians to understand the development of human embryo and more accurately select viable embryos.

In contrast to other cells (e.g., stem cells and embryonic cells of other species), automated analysis of nonstained human embryonic cells is challenged by complex development patterns such as compact growth and overlapping cells. These challenges are further complicated by the limitations of the single plane imaging limitations imposed by the dark field imaging mode, causing intensity variance and loss of depth information.

An important and first step in automated analysis is being able to efficiently and reliably segment the embryo from background noise. To this end, a framework to segment the developing embryo by estimating the contour around the embryo was developed by defining segmentation as an energy minimization problem and solving it via graph cuts [68]. Second, cells are spatially localized and divisions subsequently detected. For localization purposes, cells are modeled as ellipses fitted to the segmented outlines for each time step (**Figure 2**).

Predicting the number of cells is a fundamental task in cell biology analysis, and an indirect way to temporally locate embryo cleavage events. In the context of human embryonic cells, cell number is of prime importance as current embryo viability biomarkers require accurate cells counts. The prediction of cell numbers can either be performed directly from the microscopy images [69] or by detecting (localizing) cells [70, 71]. Both approaches can also be used in combination. In this method, a framework that combines both approaches in a conditional random field (CRF) [72] is used. The result is a model of the cell division ancestry by recording cell associations between adjacent frames, resulting in a complete lineage tree for the time-lapse sequence. Cell lineage analysis is vital in understanding dynamics of developing embryos and is a fundamental step in cell biology analysis. The cell lineage tree and segmented shapes can now be studied for various attributes of the growing embryo such as timing of cell cleavage, abnormal division patterns, and cell symmetry (**Figure 3**).

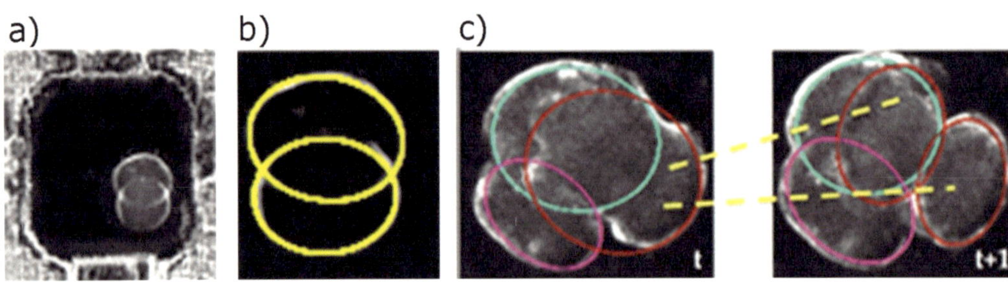

Figure 2. Example of (a) dark field microscopy image of a two-cell stage human embryo; (b) cell localization with fitted ellipses; (c) three to four cell division association for lineage tree construction.

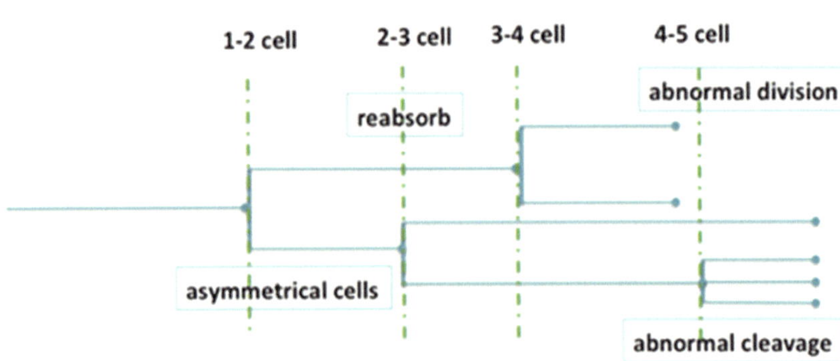

Figure 3. Proposed system for automated monitoring of early stage human embryo development.

7. Method 3: human embryo profiling using video image processing

HMC imaging is superior when it comes to image detail of human embryos. However, optical artifacts introduced by the optical modulation causes edge structures to appear with multiple gradients. Objects in focus commonly appear clearly, but at the same time, superimposed light from out-of-focus objects will often introduce "shadows" in the image. The result

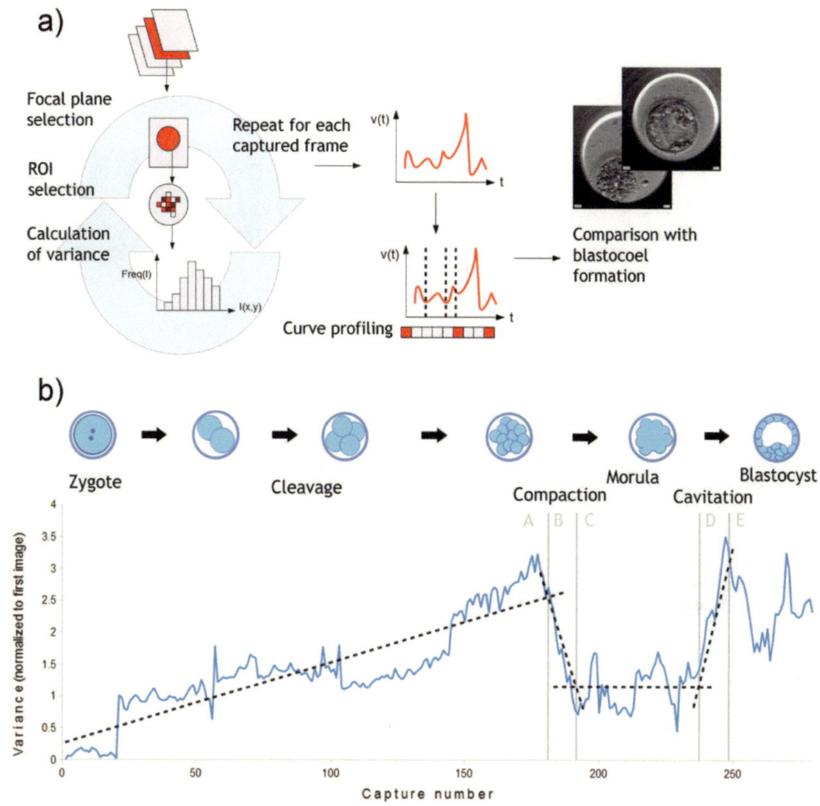

Figure 4. (a) Illustration of computational pipeline of the captured image series of an embryo. The optimal focal plane from the image stack was selected. A region of interest (ROI) was selected within each individual image, and one value of the variance in image intensity was computed for each ROI. This process was repeated for each capture in the image series, resulting in a function v(t) describing the variance as a function of time. v(t) was then further analyzed for the occurrence of detectable key events, profiling the embryo development. Finally, the profiles for embryos forming blastocysts and for those not forming blastocysts were compared. (b) Image intensity variance of an embryo during the course of 280 frame captures, normalized to the first image in the series. Divisions during the cleavage stage are detectable as sudden increases in image variance, due to the number of increased edges in the image, as blastomeres undergo mitosis. At the onset of compaction, individual blastomere membranes are no longer distinguishable, and the variance drops and remains at a low level during the morula stage. The variance increases once more as blastocoel expansion sets may fluctuate strongly during the blastocyst stage, if the embryo displays several cycles of collapse and re-expansion. The growth of the embryo has been considered in five stages. (A) Initial divisions from fertilization to onset of compaction, (B) onset to completion of compaction, (C) morula, (D) cavitation, (E) blastocyst. The mean and change in variance has been calculated for each section. Dashed trend lines have been added for illustrative purpose [75].

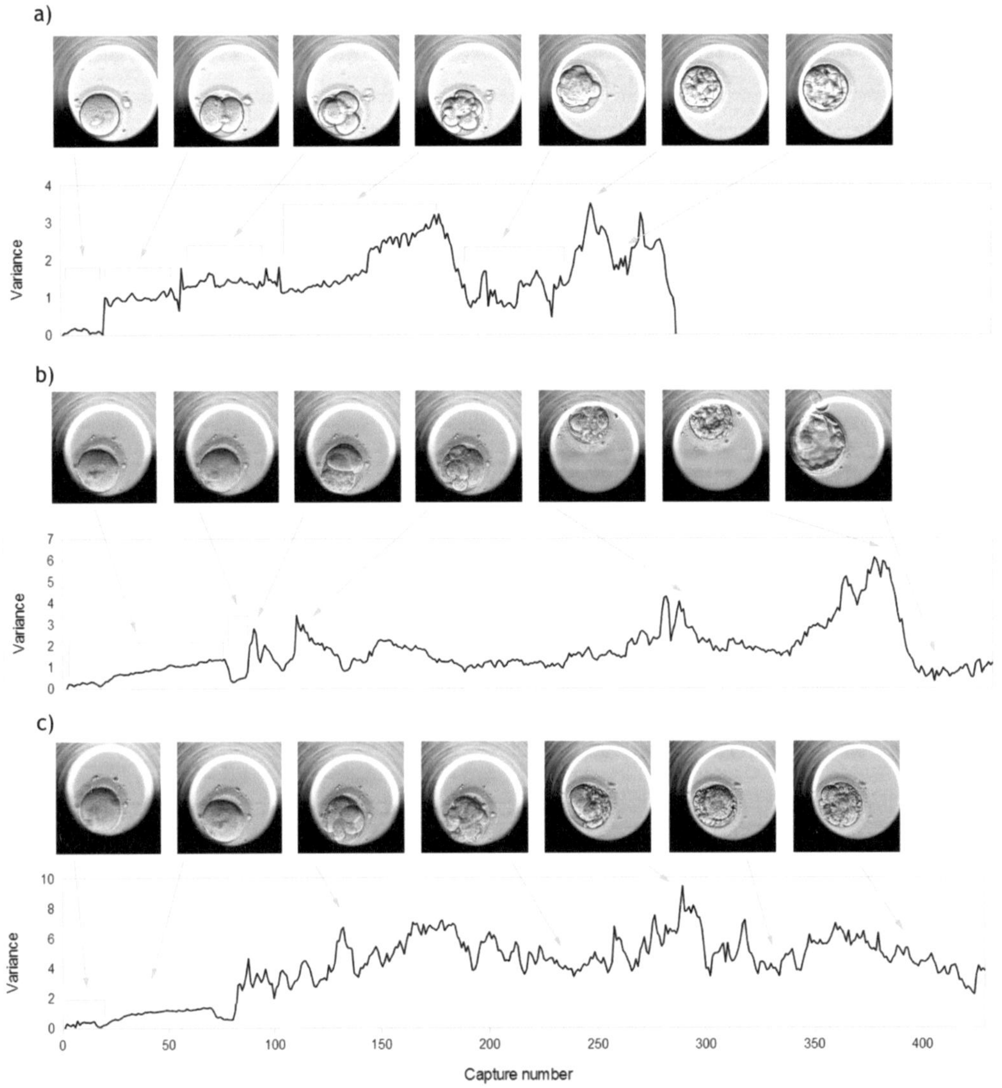

Figure 5. Profile of three representative embryos showing decreasing quality (a–c). Variance was calculated from the image intensity at a circular region encompassing the center of the embryo. A few example images are shown at points where characteristic changes are visible in the variance profile. For a good quality embryo (a) mitotic divisions are visible as successive increases in image variance, and the morula stage as a period of lowered variance; (b) illustrates a clearly expressed pronuclear breakdown, but experiences fragmentation during the cleavage stage, even though a blastocyst iseventually formed. In (c), the pronuclear breakdown is also apparent, but the embryo develops early fragments, never reaching a blastocyst stage [75].

is an image where it is inherently difficult to segment cell outlines, but with a high degree of detail in internal cell structures, despite the fact that the technique is completely marker free. Attempting to segment such an image is possible, but since subsequent analysis is often

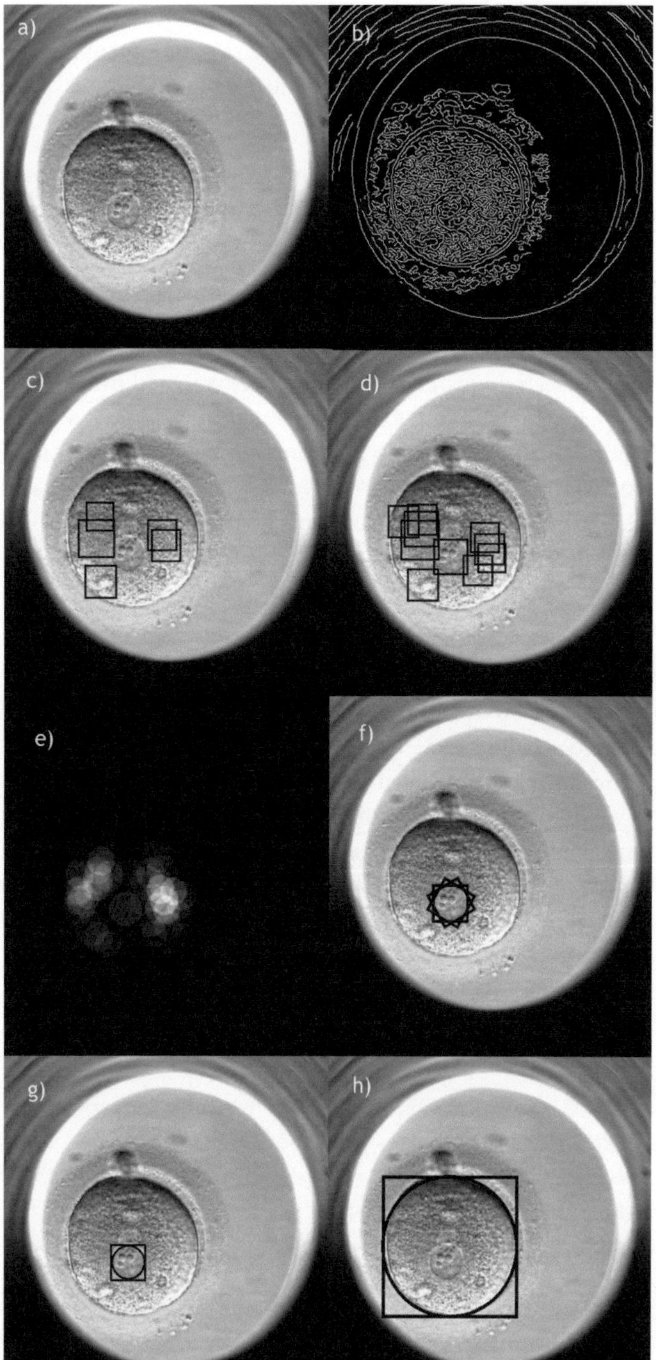

Figure 6. Detection of zygote and pronucleus in human embryo. (a) Original image. (b) Edge detection. (c) Five most significant circular structures selected. (d) 10 most significant circular structures selected. (e) Overlap of circular structures selected from the same image rotated 6 60°. (f) Outline of pronucleus indicated, overlap of three calculations at separate angles. (g) Outline of pronucleus selected. (h) Outline of zygote selected [74].

dependent on the resulting segmented outline, it is easy to introduce cumulative errors. This method focuses on the detection of developmentally relevant events in the embryo such as compaction, blastocoel formation, nuclei localization, cell cleavage, and embryo fragmentation without the need for complete segmentation.

Raw images are spatially filtered to embryo location and a set of image features are extracted from the embryo interior [73, 74]. As the embryo grows, characteristics of the image will change also the image features, making it possible to profile embryo development without the complete image data [75]. One example is shown in **Figure 4**, where the gray-level variance of the image of the embryo interior is used to plot a development sequence of the embryo in two dimensions. The gray-level variance is a measure of the contrast in the image and will increase for each cell division, as each division introduces a new cell, and thus a new set of darker cell membrane into the image, contributing to a rise in image variance. As a consequence, each cell division can be detected as a sudden steep gradient in the variance profile. The compaction is detected as a massive loss of variance as the cell membranes becomes less apparent, followed by a new increase in variance as the embryo forms a blastocoel. The ideal development of an embryo follows a predictable pattern over time, where events such as cleavage can be more easily and automatically detected than using images directly (**Figure 4**) and abnormal development will differ clearly (**Figure 5**).

Simultaneously to feature detection, segmentation of intracellular structures such as nuclei and pronuclei is possible due to the high level of image detail (**Figure 6**). The segmentation is constricted in shape and size, ensuring the located structures are of the predefined biological shape. A slight disturbance is introduced in the form of a rotation and serves to effectively average out the located structures and preventing the detection of false positives [74]. The result is a framework where the entire development from zygote to blastocyst can be profiled and combined with the visibility of relevant intracellular compartments such as nuclei, without the need for any fluorescent markers.

8. Conclusion

It has been shown that embryos can grow outside the womb for longer than 14 days, a limitation set by legal requirements [76]. This period of early embryo development has yet been little studied, due to technical constraints. New combinations of software analysis, imaging, and incubator technologies will soon make it possible to study embryo development from a whole new set of perspectives.

Using specific FP-tagged protein markers for the nucleus and plasma membrane it is possible to follow the dynamics of important morphogenetic changes during mammalian embryo development, including cell division, cell polarity, and cavitation during blastocyst formation. The quantitative analysis of these developmental hallmarks pave the way for the design of functional and phenotypical studies such as silencing (knocking down), overexpressing, or blocking using inhibitors of selected genes of interest. These method combinations can lead to the crucial understanding of developmental function and disease.

Methods for automated or semiautomated label-free analysis of embryos in vivo make it possible to study embryo development over longer times than previously possible—opening up a new set of insights into especially early human development, where ethical considerations are important for the choice of study method. By time-lapse sequence studies of routinely growing embryos in IVF, the research data can be gathered in a clinical context, and methods can simultaneously contribute to better IVF embryo monitoring.

In conclusion, these noninvasive methods open a window to increase the understanding of general developmental embryology as well as specific medical questions such as embryo division patterns, lineage, and the reasons behind the low human fertility rates.

Acknowledgements

Anna Leida Mölder is grateful for the help and support of Manchester Metropolitan University. Juan Carlos Fierro-González is grateful for the support received from the Swedish Society for Medical Research.

Author details

Anna Leida Mölder[1]*, Juan Carlos Fierro-González[2] and Aisha Khan[3]

*Address all correspondence to: mail@annaleida.com

1 Manchester Metropolitan University, Manchester, UK

2 Chalmers University of Technology, Department of Biology and Biological Engineering, Gothenburg, Sweden

3 Research & Engineering, Progyny Inc, New York, USA

References

[1] Diamond MP, Willman S, Chenette P, Cedars MI. The clinical need for a method of identification of embryos destined to become a blastocyst in assisted reproductive technology cycles. Journal of Assisted Reproduction and Genetics. 2012 May 1;**29**(5):391-396

[2] Kupka MS, D'Hooghe T, Ferraretti AP, Mouzon de J, et al. Assisted reproductive technology in Europe, 2011: Results generated from European registers by ESHRE. Human Reproduction. 2016 Feb 1;**31**(2):233-248

[3] Hardarson T, Ahlström A, Rogberg L, Botros L, Hillensjö T, Westlander G, et al. Non-invasive metabolomic profiling of Day 2 and 5 embryo culture medium: A prospective randomized trial. Human Reproduction (Oxford, England). 2012 Jan 1;**27**(1):89-96

[4] Mastenbroek S, Twisk M, van Echten-Arends J, Sikkema-Raddatz B, Korevaar JC, Verhoeve HR, et al. In vitro fertilization with preimplantation genetic screening. New England Journal of Medicine. 2007 Jul 5;**357**(1):9-17

[5] Vergouw CG, Kieslinger DC, Kostelijk EH, Hompes PG, Schats R, Lambalk CB. Metabolomic profiling of culture media by near-infrared spectroscopy as an adjunct to morphology for selection of a single day 3 embryo to transfer in IVF: A double-blind randomised trial. Fertility and Sterility. 2011 Sep 1;**96**(3):S3

[6] Ottosen LDM, Hindkjaer J, Ingerslev J. Light exposure of the ovum and preimplantation embryo during ART procedures. Journal of Assisted Reproduction and Genetics. 2007 Mar;**24**(2-3):99-103

[7] Jones GM, Cram DS, Song B, Kokkali G, Pantos K, Trounson AO. Novel strategy with potential to identify developmentally competent IVF blastocysts. Human Reproduction (Oxford, England). 2008 Aug;**23**(8):1748-1759

[8] Scott L, Berntsen J, Davies D, Gundersen J, Hill J, Ramsing N. Symposium: Innovative techniques in human embryo viability assessment. Human oocyte respiration-rate measurement—potential to improve oocyte and embryo selection? Reproductive Biomedicine Online. 2008 Oct;**17**(4):461-469

[9] Seli E, Robert C, Sirard M-A. OMICS in assisted reproduction: Possibilities and pitfalls. Molecular Human Reproduction. 2010 Aug;**16**(8):513-530

[10] Hardarson T, Caisander G, Sjögren A, Hanson C, Hamberger L, Lundin K. A morphological and chromosomal study of blastocysts developing from morphologically suboptimal human pre-embryos compared with control blastocysts. Human Reproduction (Oxford, England). 2003 Feb;**18**(2):399-407

[11] Montag M, Liebenthron J, Köster M. Which morphological scoring system is relevant in human embryo development? Placenta. 2011 Sep;**32**(Suppl 3):S252-S256

[12] Van Blerkom J, Davis P, Alexander S. A microscopic and biochemical study of fragmentation phenotypes in stage-appropriate human embryos. Human Reproduction (Oxford, England). 2001 Apr;**16**(4):719-729

[13] Lemmen JG, Agerholm I, Ziebe S. Kinetic markers of human embryo quality using time-lapse recordings of IVF/ICSI-fertilized oocytes. Reproductive Biomedicine Online. 2008 Sep;**17**(3):385-391

[14] Alikani M, Cohen J, Tomkin G, Garrisi GJ, Mack C, Scott RT. Human embryo fragmentation in vitro and its implications for pregnancy and implantation. Fertility and Sterility. 1999 May;**71**(5):836-842

[15] Cruz M, Garrido N, Herrero J, Pérez-Cano I, Muñoz M, Meseguer M. Timing of cell division in human cleavage-stage embryos is linked with blastocyst formation and quality. Reproductive Biomedicine Online. 2012 Oct;**25**(4):371-381

[16] Chen AA, Tan L, Suraj V, Reijo Pera R, Shen S. Biomarkers identified with time-lapse imaging: Discovery, validation, and practical application. Fertility and Sterility. 2013 Mar 15;**99**(4):1035-1043

[17] Hlinka D, Kaľatová B, Uhrinová I, Dolinská S, Rutarová J, Rezáčová J, et al. Time-lapse cleavage rating predicts human embryo viability. Physiological Research. 2012; **61**(5):513-525

[18] Meseguer M, Herrero J, Tejera A, Hilligsøe KM, Ramsing NB, Remohí J. The use of morphokinetics as a predictor of embryo implantation. Human Reproduction (Oxford, England). 2011 Oct;**26**(10):2658-2671

[19] Sato S, Rancourt A, Sato Y, Satoh MS. Single-cell lineage tracking analysis reveals that an established cell line comprises putative cancer stem cells and their heterogeneous progeny. Scientific Report. 2016;**6**: 23328. PubMed: 27003384

[20] Van Valen DA, Kudo T, Lane KM, Macklin DN, Quach NT, DeFelice MM, et al. Deep learning automates the quantitative analysis of individual cells in live-cell imaging experiments. PLoS Computational Biology. 2016 Nov;**12**(11):e1005177

[21] Llamosi A, Gonzalez-Vargas AM, Versari C, Cinquemani E, Ferrari-Trecate G, Hersen P, et al. What population reveals about individual cell identity: Single-cell parameter estimation of models of gene expression in yeast. PLoS Computational Biology. 2016; **12**(2):e1004706

[22] Merouane A, Rey-Villamizar N, Lu Y, Liadi I, Romain G, Lu J, et al. Automated profiling of individual cell-cell interactions from high-throughput time-lapse imaging microscopy in nanowell grids (TIMING). Bioinformatics (Oxford, England). 2015 Oct 1;**31**(19):3189-3197

[23] Combs CA. Fluorescence microscopy: A concise guide to current imaging methods. Current Protocols in Neuroscience. 2010;2.1

[24] Stephens DJ, Allan VJ. Light microscopy techniques for live cell imaging. Science. 2003;**300**(5616):82-86. PubMed: 12677057

[25] Chalfie M, et al. Green fluorescent protein as a marker for gene expression. Science. 1994;**263**(5148):802-805. PubMed: 8303295

[26] Shimomura O, Johnson FH, Saiga Y. Extraction, purification and properties of aequorin, a bioluminescent protein from the luminous hydromedusan, Aequorea. Journal of Cellular and Comparative Physiology. 1962;**59**:223-239. PubMed: 13911999

[27] Magidson V, Khodjakov A. Circumventing photodamage in live-cell microscopy. Methods in Cell Biology. 2013;**114**:545-560

[28] White J, Stelzer E. Photobleaching GFP reveals protein dynamics inside live cells. Trends in Cell Biology. 1999;**9**(2):61-65. PubMed: 10087620

[29] Miyawaki A. Proteins on the move: Insights gained from fluorescent protein technologies. Nature Reviews Molecular Cell Biology. 2011 Sep 23;**12**(10):656-668

[30] Kenworthy AK. Imaging protein-protein interactions using fluorescence resonance energy transfer microscopy. Methods (San Diego, Calif.). 2001 Jul;**24**(3):289-296

[31] Plachta N, Bollenbach T, Pease S, Fraser SE, Pantazis P. Oct4 kinetics predict cell lineage patterning in the early mammalian embryo. Nature Cell Biology. 2011 Feb;**13**(2):117-123

[32] Fierro-González JC, White MD, Silva JC, Plachta N. Cadherin-dependent filopodia control preimplantation embryo compaction. Nature Cell Biology. 2013;**15**:(1424-1433)

[33] White MD, Angiolini JF, Alvarez YD, Kaur G, Zhao ZW, Mocskos E, et al. Long-lived binding of Sox2 to DNA predicts cell fate in the four-cell mouse embryo. Cell. 2016 Mar 24;**165**(1):75-87

[34] Kaur G, Costa MW, Nefzger CM, Silva J, Fierro-González JC, Polo JM, et al. Probing transcription factor diffusion dynamics in the living mammalian embryo with photoactivatable fluorescence correlation spectroscopy. Nature Communications. 2013 Mar 27;**4**:1637

[35] Boxman J, Sagy N, Achanta S, Vadigepalli R, Nachman I. Integrated live imaging and molecular profiling of embryoid bodies reveals a synchronized progression of early differentiation. Scientific Reports 2016 Aug 17;**6**:31623

[36] Chen J, Zhang Z, Li L, Chen B-C, Revyakin A, Hajj B, et al. Single-molecule dynamics of enhanceosome assembly in embryonic stem cells. Cell. 2014 Mar 13;**156**(6):1274-1285

[37] Embryoscope Time-Lapse System [Internet]. http://www.vitrolife.com/sv/Products/EmbryoScope-Time-Lapse-System/ [Accessed: January 17, 2017]

[38] Primo Vision Time-Lapse System [Internet]. http://www.vitrolife.com/en/Fertility/Products/Primo-Vision-Time-Lapse-System/ [Accessed: January 17, 2017]

[39] Eeva [Internet]. https://www.eevatest.com/ [Accessed: January 17, 2017]

[40] Evans CL, Xie XS. Coherent anti-stokes Raman scattering microscopy: Chemical imaging for biology and medicine. Annual Review of Analytical Chemistry (Palo Alto, California). 2008;**1**:883-909

[41] Tomer R, Khairy K, Keller PJ. Light sheet microscopy in cell biology. Methods (San Diego, Calif.). 2013;**931**:123-137

[42] Pluta M. Advanced Light Microscopy (3 Vols.). New York: Elsevier, 1989; **1**:464, **2**:494, **3**:702

[43] Hoffman R. The modulation contrast microscope: Principles and performance. Journal of Microscopy. 1977;**110**(3):205-222

[44] Kovacs P. Embryo selection: The role of time-lapse monitoring. Reproductive Biology and Endocrinology: RBE. 2014; **12**:**124**

[45] Polanski LT, Coelho Neto MA, Nastri CO, Navarro PA, Ferriani RA, Raine-Fenning N, et al. Time-lapse embryo imaging for improving reproductive outcomes: Systematic review and meta-analysis. Ultrasound in Obstetrics and Gynecology. 2014 Oct 1;**44**(4):394-401

[46] Kahraman S, Çetinkaya M, Pirkevi C, Yelke H, Kumtepe Y. Comparison of blastocyst development and cycle outcome in patients with eSET using either conventional or time lapse incubators. A prospective study of good prognosis patients. Journal of Reproductive and Stem Cell Biotechnology. 2012 Dec 1;**3**(2):55-61

[47] Kirkegaard K, Hindkjaer JJ, Grøndahl ML, Kesmodel US, Ingerslev HJ. A randomized clinical trial comparing embryo culture in a conventional incubator with a time-lapse incubator. Journal of Assisted Reproduction and Genetics. 2012 Jun;**29**(6):565-572

[48] Park H, Bergh C, Selleskog U, Thurin-Kjellberg A, Lundin K. No benefit of culturing embryos in a closed system compared with a conventional incubator in terms of number of good quality embryos: Results from an RCT. Human Reproduction (Oxford, England). 2015 Feb;**30**(2):268-275

[49] Paternot G, Wetzels AM, Thonon F, Vansteenbrugge A, Willemen D, Devroe J, et al. Intra- and interobserver analysis in the morphological assessment of early stage embryos during an IVF procedure: A multicentre study. Reproductive Biology and Endocrinology. 2011;**9**:127

[50] Sundvall L, Ingerslev HJ, Knudsen UB, Kirkegaard K. Inter- and intra-observer variability of time-lapse annotations. Human Reproduction (Oxford, England). 2013 Sep 26;**2013**(28):3215-3221

[51] Allan C, Burel J-M, Moore J, Blackburn C, Linkert M, Loynton S, et al. OMERO: Flexible, model-driven data management for experimental biology. Nature Methods. 2012 Feb 28;**9**(3):245-253

[52] Beuchat A, Thévenaz P, Unser M, Ebner T, Senn A, Urner F, et al. Quantitative morphometrical characterization of human pronuclear zygotes. Human Reproduction (Oxford, England). 2008 Sep;**23**(9):1983-1992

[53] Filho ES, Noble J., Wells D. A review on automatic analysis of human embryo microscope images. Open Biomedical Engineering Journal. 2010 Oct 11;**4**:170-177

[54] Giusti A, Corani G, Gambardella LM, Magli MC, Gianaroli L. Blastomere segmentation and 3D morphology measurements of early embryos from Hoffman Modulation Contrast image stacks. In: 2010 IEEE International Symposium on Biomedical Imaging: From Nano to Macro. 2010;1261-1264

[55] Wong CC, Loewke KE, Bossert NL, Behr B, De Jonge CJ, Baer TM, et al. Non-invasive imaging of human embryos before embryonic genome activation predicts development to the blastocyst stage. Nature Biotechnology. 2010 Oktober;**28**(10):1115-1121

[56] Moussavi F, Wang Y, Lorenzen P, Oakley J, Russakoff D, Gould S. A unified graphical models framework for automated mitosis detection in human embryos. IEEE Transactions on Medical Imaging. 2014 Jul;**33**(7):1551-1562

[57] Agerholm IE, Hnida C, Cruger DG, Berg C, Bruun-Petersen G, Kølvraa S, et al. Nuclei size in relation to nuclear status and aneuploidy rate for 13 chromosomes in donated four cells embryos. Journal of Assisted Reproduction and Genetics. 2008 Mar;**25**(2-3):95-102

[58] Morales DA, Bengoetxea E, Larranaga P. Automatic segmentation of zona pellucida in human embryo images applying an active contour model. In: Proc 12th Annu Conf Med Image Underst Anal. 2008:209-213

[59] Filho ES, Noble JA, Poli M, Griffiths T, Emerson G, Wells D. A method for semi-automatic grading of human blastocyst microscope images. Human Reproduction (Oxford, England). 2012 Sep;**27**(9):2641-2648

[60] Kang M, Xenopoulos P, Muñoz-Descalzo S, Lou X, Hadjantonakis A-K. Live imaging, identifying, and tracking single cells in complex populations in vivo and ex vivo. Methods in Molecular Biology (Clifto, NJ). 2013;**1052**:109-123

[61] Turksen K. Imaging and tracking stem cells : Methods and protocols. NY, USA: New York Humana Press; 2013

[62] Tsien RY. The green fluorescent protein. Annual Review of Biochemistry. 1998;**67**(509-544)

[63] Fine A. Confocal microscopy: Principles and practice. Chapter 6, Yuste R & Konnerth A editors. In Imaging in Neuroscience and Development. NY, USA: Cold Spring Harbor Laboratory Press, Cold Spring Harbor; 2005

[64] Ustione A, Piston DW. A simple introduction to multiphoton microscopy. Journal of Microscopy. 2011 Sep;**243**(3):221-226

[65] Samarage CR, White MD, Alvarez YD, Fierro-Gonzalez JC, Henon Y, Jesudason EC, Bissiere S, Fouras A, Plachta N. Cortical tension allocates the first inner cells of the mammalian embryo. Developmental Cell. 2015;**34**:435-447

[66] Turner DL, Weintraub H. Expression of achaete-scute homolog 3 in Xenopus embryos converts ectodermal cells to a neural fate. Genes and Development. 1994;**8**:1434-1447

[67] Louvet-Vallee S, Dard N, Santa-Maria A, Aghion J, Maro B. A major posttranslational modification of ezrin takes place during epithelial differentiation in the early mouse embryo. Developments in Biologicals. 2001;**231**:190-200

[68] Khan A, Gould S and Salzmann M. Segmentation of developing human embryo in time-lapse microscopy. In: Proc. IEEE International Symposium on Biomedical Imaging; 2016

[69] Khan A, Gould S, and Salzmann M. Automated monitoring of human embryonic cells up to the 5-cell stage in time-lapse microscopy images. In: Proc. 12th IEEE International Symposium on Biomedical Imaging; 2015

[70] Khan A, Gould S, and Salzmann M. A linear chain Markov model for detection and localization of cells in early stage embryo development. In: Winter Conference on Applications of Computer Vision; 2015:526-533

[71] Khan A, Gould S and Salzmann M. Deep convolutional neural networks for human embryonic cell counting. In: Workshop on Bioimage Computing at European Conference on Computer Vision; 2016:339-348

http://dx.doi.org/10.5772/intechopen.69650

[72] Khan A, Gould S, and Salzmann M. Detecting abnormal cell division patterns in early stage human embryo development. In 6th International Workshop on Machine Learning in Medical Imaging; 2015:161-169

[73] Mölder A, Drury S, Costen N, Hartshorne GM, Czanner S. Semiautomated analysis of embryoscope images: Using localized variance of image intensity to detect embryo developmental stages. Cytometry. Part A. 2015 Feb 1;**87**(2):119-128

[74] Mölder A, Czanner S, Costen N, Hartshorne G. Automatic detection of circular structures in human embryo imaging using trigonometric rotation of the Hough Transform. In: 22nd International Conference on Pattern Recognition (ICPR). 2014:3239-3244

[75] Deglincerti A, Croft GF, Pietila LN, Zernicka-Goetz M, Siggia ED, Brivanlou AH. Self-organization of the in vitro attached human embryo. Nature. 2016 Mar;**533**(7602):251-254

[76] Mölder A, Czanner S, Costen N. Focal plane selection in microscopic embryo images. In: Conference on Computer Graphics & Visual Computing; 2014

Section 3

Gene Expression of Cleavage Embryo and Non-invasive Assessment

Chapter 5

Control of Embryonic Gene Expression and Epigenetics

Pinar Tulay

Additional information is available at the end of the chapter

http://dx.doi.org/10.5772/67851

Abstract

Preimplantation embryo development follows a series of critical events. Remarkable epigenetic modifications and reprogramming of gene expression occur to activate the embryonic genome. In the early stages of preimplantation embryo development, maternal mRNAs direct embryonic development. Throughout early embryonic development, a differential methylation pattern is maintained although some show stage-specific changes. Recent studies have shown that differential demethylation process results in differential parental gene expression in the early developing embryos that may have an impact on the correct development. In the recent years, noncoding RNAs, long noncoding RNAs (lncRNA) and short of mRNAs and therefore their role in preimplantation development has gained significance.

Keywords: gene expression, methylation, miRNA

1. Introduction

Preimplantation embryo development follows a series of critical events. These events start at gametogenesis, formation of mature gametes, and lasts until parturition. Male and female gametes are derived from primordial germ cells (PGCs) by the processes of spermatogenesis and oogenesis, respectively. PGCs have unique properties of gene expression, epigenetics, morphology and behaviour. Once the PGCs undergo mitosis, spermatogenesis and oogenesis progress differently. In spermatogenesis, spermatogonia undergo mitosis starting at puberty until death and each primary spermatocyte produces four spermatids at the end of meiosis. In oogenesis, PGCs differentiate into oogonia, they enter meiosis and arrest until puberty. Unlike meiosis II in spermatogenesis, secondary oocyte does not complete meiosis II until fertilisation. With completion of meiosis II, each oogonia produce a single viable oocyte [1].

At fertilisation, the oocyte completes meiosis and the fertilised oocyte is called the zygote. Oocyte and sperm nuclei fuse resulting in syngamy (**Figure 1**). The zygote undergoes a series of cleavage divisions, forming two-cell, four-cell, eight-cell morula and blastocyst stages [2] (**Figure 1**). During cleavage stage divisions, programming of maternal and paternal chromosomes takes place to create the embryonic genome (embryonic genome activation, EGA) and to start the preimplantation embryo development. If the EGA fails, the development does not continue because of the inability of the embryo to have cellular functions [3]. This activation is initiated by the degradation of maternal nucleic acids, specific RNAs stored in oocytes, proteins and other macromolecules [4]. Upon EGA, which starts at the two-cell stage in mouse and four- to eight-cell stage in human [5], remarkable reprogramming of expression occurs in the preimplantation embryo. These reprogramming events are controlled by DNA methylation, histone acetylation, transcription, translation and miRNA regulation [6]. Therefore, the development of preimplantation embryos includes continuous molecular, cellular and morphological events. These events would eventually form a multilineage embryo that has a capability to implant and continue the foetal development.

In this chapter, different factors affecting gene expression during preimplantation embryo development will be discussed. Epigenetic factors, focusing on methylation profiles, of gametes and preimplantation embryos will be reviewed. The effects of noncoding RNAs on gene expression will be thoroughly evaluated.

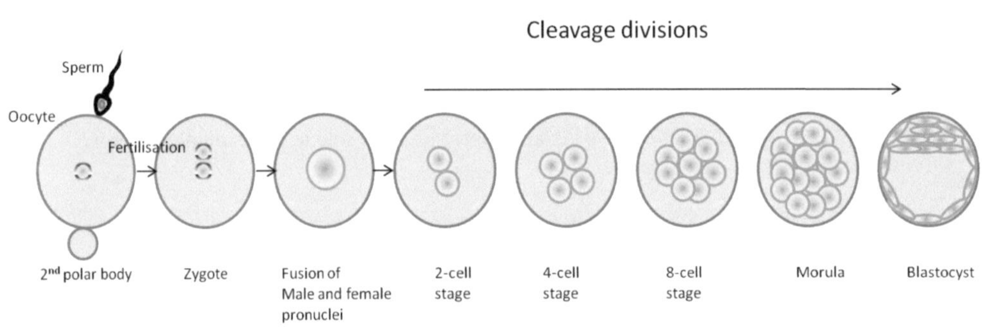

Figure 1. Schematic diagram outlining the main stages of preimplantation embryo development. Fertilisation followed by syngamy, cleavage divisions results in two, three, four, and so on cell embryos which eventually form the morula and the blastocyst.

2. Gene expression and epigenetics

For a normal developing embryo, the expression of both maternal and paternal genes is required. An intense epigenetic change occurs upon fertilisation to establish pluripotency [7]. Although there are a number of post-translational modifications within chromatin including acetylation, ubiquitination, SUMOylation and phosphorylation; methylation of histone lysine and arginine residues is the main focus in preimplantation embryos.

Methylation and chromatin modification not only play crucial roles in determining the transcriptional state but also are capable of determining the transcriptional repression

[8–10]. The mechanism leading to the changes in methylation is not well established, but it has been suggested that the reprogramming takes place by either passive or active demethylation. Indirect pathways of demethylation are associated with DNA repair [11–14]. Two main stages, PGCs and preimplantation embryos, are important in the regulation by methylation.

2.1. Epigenetic modification of the zygote and the preimplantation embryos

In mammals (human, bovine, rat, pig and mouse), the zygote undergoes genome-wide demethylation [15–17] with the exception of imprinted genes [18]. The male pronucleus of the zygote undergoes selective demethylation due to the loss of DNA replication leading to asymmetric methylated sister chromatids [15, 16, 19, 20]. These events start following the sperm decondensation in humans and in mouse with some variations [17, 21, 22]. The female pronucleus of the zygote remains highly methylated at this stage [17, 21, 22]. Demethylation of the maternal genome starts with the first cleavage divisions [19, 23, 24]. By the morula stage, the mouse preimplantation embryos become undermethylated. Polarisation and compaction of individual blastomeres start at around eight-cell stage of the developing embryo. Many factors are involved in these processes including E-cadherin (CDH1), partitioning defective homologue 3 (PARD3), PARD6B and protein kinase C zeta [25–27].

The blastocyst stage embryo has a fluid-filled cavity and two cell populations consisting of inner cell mass (ICM) and trophectoderm (TE). All the blastomeres are believed to be totipotent in cleavage embryos until four- to eight-cell stage since these cells form both the ICM and TE lineage [28]. ICM develops into epiblast, whereas TE forms the extraembryonic tissues such as placenta. ICM is composed of pluripotent cells that have the capacity to develop into any cell type of the foetus. Transcriptional and epigenetic events strictly regulate these differentiation events. A number of transcriptional factors play a crucial role in blastocyst formation. These include caudal type homeobox 2 (CDX2) for TE specification, octamer 3/4 (OCT4) and NANOG for the establishment of ICM pluripotency [29–31]. CDX2 is extensively expressed in eight- and 16-cell stage and it is expressed only in TE cells of the blastocyst [32]. Although OCT4 and NANOG are also expressed broadly at eight- and 16-cell stage embryos, they are only expressed in ICM in blastocysts [32]. A number of transcription factors are required for blastocyst formation. Embryos lacking CDX2 expression cannot form blastocoel cavity but they have the ability to implant [30]. Lack of OCT4 or NANOG expression causes failure of ICM and the development of these embryos is arrested at the blastocyst stage [31, 32]. TEAD4 is another transcription factor that has a role in blastocyst transition in which the lack of TEAD4 nuclear localisation impairs TE-specific transcriptional programme in inner blastomeres [33]. Furthermore, the aberrant expression of TCFAP2C transcription factor also leads to embryonic arrest during morula to blastocyst transition [34] and Klf5 mouse-mutant embryos arrest at the blastocyst stage [35].

The remethylation process starts shortly after implantation [16, 22, 23, 36]. This *de novo* methylation occurs asymmetrically, such that ICM is hypermethylated possibly due to the Dnmt3b methylase [37], whereas TE remains hypomethylated due to the active demethylation by enzyme catalysis and passive demethylation [11, 14, 22]. Alteration of the methylation profiles in embryos has been shown to cause alterations of ICM and TE differentiation.

Variations of the H3 arginine 26 residue (H3R26me) were shown to lead to changes of TE and ICM differentiation of a blastomere [38].

X-chromosome inactivation is an epigenetic phenomenon in which the activity of X chromosomes is strictly regulated to equalise X-chromosome expression and gene dosage between males and females and relative to autosome chromosomes [39]. For correct development, X-chromosome dosage compensation is crucial. The inactivation of X chromosome occurs in at least two phases: initiation and maintenance. X-inactivation mouse model systems have shown that the inactivation of X chromosome takes place during early embryogenesis of the female embryo by undergoing transcriptional silencing of genes along the X chromosome [40]. In human preimplantation embryos, it has been shown that the reduced expression of X chromosomes in females ensures the dosage compensation [41]. LncRNA *XIST* expression activates the X-chromosome inactivation by engaging proteins functioning in chromatin remodelling [3, 42]. With the advanced technologies, including single-cell RNA sequencing, it has emerged that lncRNAs *XACT* and *XIST* are expressed on the active X chromosome in the early human preimplantation embryos [43]. Furthermore, the expression of these two RNAs has never been shown to overlap. Introducing *XACT* into heterologous systems caused the accumulation of *Xist* RNA in *cis* and therefore it may be involved in the control of *XIST* association to chromosome in *cis* and may temper its ability of silencing. It is also possible that *XACT* functions in balancing the X-chromosome inactivation at the early stages of preimplantation embryo development [43, 44]. Recently, the dosage compensation was shown to be driven by a CAG promoter of a new Xist allele (Xist(CAG)) [45]. Furthermore, Xist(CAG) upregulation in preimplantation embryos showed variation depending on the parental origin and the paternal expression was suggested to be preferentially inactivated with the paternal Xist(CAG) transmission [45].

2.2. Epigenetic modification of the gametes

In germ cells, methylation is maintained in a sex-specific manner. Methylation in PGCs diminishes as they migrate to the gonads. Studies suggest that in females, remethylation occurs after birth when the oocytes are in the process of development. When demethylation is completed, the PGCs either enter mitosis in males or arrest at meiosis in females [46].

Reprogramming of the methylation in the embryo is necessary for parent-specific expression of genes [14]. Gene expression varies during preimplantation embryo development due to these reprogramming events and appropriate gene expression determines the survival of the embryo [6]. Recently, short noncoding RNAs, microRNAs (miRNAs) and long noncoding RNAs (lncRNA) have gained importance in their potential function to affect numerous pathways by targeting multiple genes [47, 48].

3. Gene expression and small noncoding RNAs: microRNAs

MiRNAs are a large family of short noncoding RNAs between 17 and 25 nucleotides (nt) in length [49]. MiRNAs were first identified in *Caenorhabditis elegans* over two decades ago

[50] and since then many have been identified in multiple organisms, such as worms, flies, fish, frogs, mammals and plants, by molecular cloning and bioinformatics [51]. Most miRNA sequences are conserved among a wide range of mammalians [52], though there are some that differ from each other only by a single nucleotide [53]. The conserved miRNA sequences among different species can be distinguished by the nomenclature such that when only the first three letters differ this indicates the same sequence in different species, that is, hsa-miR-145 in *Homo sapiens* and mmu-miR-145 in *Mus musculus* [54].

MiRNAs have been shown to be of great importance in a wide variety of biological processes involving cell cycle regulation, apoptosis, cell differentiation, imprinting, homeostasis and development, including limb development [55], morphogenesis of lung epithelial [56], embryonic angiogenesis [57], formation of hair follicle and proliferation of T-cell [58, 59]. They play key roles in regulating transcriptional and post-transcriptional gene silencing in many organisms by targeting mRNAs for translational inhibition, cleavage, degradation or destabilisation [53, 60–64]. Each miRNA has multiple mRNA targets that may regulate up to 30% protein-coding genes and shape protein production from hundreds to thousands of genes [65–67]. MiRNAs recognise their targets through base pairing of the complementary sequence of their seed sequence (2–8 nt of miRNAs) within the open reading frame (ORF) and 3'untranslated region (UTR) of target mRNA [68]. Although the targets of miRNAs are not fully known, bioinformatics studies show a range of possible target genes [69]. The functional activities and the predicted/observed targets of miRNAs can be identified using miRNA databases. These databases can be accessed using the following URL: (http://www.targetscan.org/, http://www.microrna.org/microrna/home.do and http://mirdb.org/miRDB/).

3.1. MiRNA biogenesis

MiRNA biogenesis involves multiple important steps. MiRNAs are first transcribed from genomic DNA into primary miRNA (pri-miRNA), which contains a stem-loop structure, by RNA polymerase II. These pri-miRNAs are then processed by Drosha, which is a 30–160 kDa protein with one dsRNA-binding and two catalytic domains [70]. In the presence of DGCR8, both strands of the hairpin are cut generating a pre-miRNA product of approximately 70 nt in size [71]. These pre-miRNAs are carried from the nucleus into the cytoplasm by Exportin-5 (Exp5), which is a nucleocytoplasmic transporter in karyopherin family that has binding sites for pre-miRNAs in the presence of RAs-related nuclear protein (Ran) and guanosine triphosphate (GTP) [72, 73]. These miRNAs are further cleaved by cytoplasmic RNase endonuclease, Dicer, making 21–22 nt double-stranded structure. Although one of the strands is usually degraded, both strands of the pre-miRNA may be associated with Argonaute (Ago)-protein-containing complex and they are mediated by RISC/miRNP (RNA-induced silencing complex/mi-ribonucleoprotein) to form single-stranded mature miRNAs. MiRNAs associated with RISC mainly target mRNAs and they either inhibit their translation or cause degradation of mRNA that results in reduced protein synthesis [70, 74].

Studies showed that processing of miRNAs by Dicer was vital and any defects, such as deletion of Dicer in the developing animals, caused aberrations [75, 76]. Lack of Dicer in Drosophila germ line stem cells postponed the G1/S phase transition [77], suggesting that miRNAs may be vital for stem cells to bypass this checkpoint. Reduced and disorganised spindles, incorrect chromosome alignment and defects in gastrulation were observed with the Dicer-mutant oocytes in mouse and in *C. elegans*, respectively [50, 78]. Injection of miR-430 in zebrafish and *C. elegans* partially repaired the gastrulation, retinal development and somatogenesis [78]. Dicer deletion in zebrafish, mouse and hippocampal initiated problems in the nervous system and led to the inability of forming mature miRNAs that resulted in variations of brain morphogenesis and differentiation of neurons [79, 80]. Although the axis formation and early differentiation of maternal-zygotic Dicer-mutant zebrafish and mouse embryos were normal, they still triggered defects in somitogenesis, morphogenesis that affected the brain formation, gastrulation, heart development and apoptosis in limb mesoderm, respectively [78, 81–83]. Apoptosis was enhanced in the developing limb mesoderm of Dicer null mouse [84]. Dicer deficiency mainly led to embryo death in mouse around embryonic day 7.5 [50, 78, 85] and in zebrafish [86] that may indicate the importance of miRNA-mediated gene silencing at maternal to zygotic transition.

Complete loss of Dicer1 in somatic cells of mouse reproductive tract not only showed reduced expression of miRNAs but also caused the female mice to become infertile with compromised oocyte and embryo integrity [50, 87]. Dicer-deficient male mice were shown to have poor proliferation of spermatogonia. Loss of Dicer1 in the germ line of male mice (homozygote Dicer1) led to decreased fertility due to abnormal spermatogenesis. The number of germ cells was reduced with abnormal spermatids, abnormal phenotype of spermatocytes with condensed nucleus, abnormal sperm motility and mutant testes with Sertoli tubules [88]. Studies suggest that the transfer of maternal cytoplasmic Dicer disguised the early abnormal phenotypes [78, 89].

Knock-out of Ago2 in mouse embryonic fibroblasts and haematopoietic cells caused decreased levels of mature miRNAs [61, 90, 91]. Ago2-deficient oocytes were observed to develop the mature oocytes with abnormal spindles and chromosomes were not able to unite properly with reduced expression levels of miRNAs (more than 80%). Loss of Ago2 function leads to embryo death around embryonic day 9.5 in mouse [92].

3.2. Expression of miRNAs in preimplantation embryos

The expression of miRNAs in preimplantation embryos has been mainly studied by knock-out experiments, by cloning experiments and by identifying individual miRNAs by microarray analysis and real-time polymerase chain reaction [93]. The expression studies have been carried out using animal models and tissues, cultured cells; that is, cancer cells and human embryonic stem cells; and mouse/bovine/human gametes and embryos. Human embryonic stem cells, which are derived from the inner cell mass of an embryo at the blastocyst stage and are characterised by their ability of self-renewal and multipotency, are the key in gene expression research since the access of human embryos is difficult and these cells are one of the closest representations of human embryos. Studying miRNA expression in stem cells not only gives insight into potential miRNAs expressed in human embryos but also may show the important role of miRNAs in the stem cell functioning [94].

MiRNA expression has been observed as early as oogenesis and spermatogenesis in mouse, bovine and human [95, 96]. Differences in the miRNA expression have been observed between

http://dx.doi.org/10.5772/67851

immature and mature oocytes that may represent the natural turnover and indicate that each embryonic stage is defined by a specific miRNA. Similar miRNA expression profiles in mature mouse oocytes and early developing embryos indicate that at these stages the zygote has maternally inherited miRNAs [50]. Similar to oocyte, sperm carries a range of miRNAs. Approximately 20% of these miRNAs are located in the nuclear or perinuclear part of the sperm indicating that these miRNAs are transferred to the zygote at the time of fertilisation [97]. It was suggested that the sperm-borne miRNAs may down-regulate the maternal transcripts in mammals. However, when this hypothesis was tested using microarray analysis, it was shown that none of these miRNAs in the sperm have significant importance since all of them were already present in the oocytes (meiosis II) [98].

Multiple miRNAs were involved in the formation of germ cell layers. MiR-290, which was expressed at different levels during preimplantation embryo development of mouse embryos, had a negative effect on the germ cell and mesoderm differentiation in the mouse ES cells *via* targeting Nodal inhibitors [99]. In zebrafish, however, miR-290 cluster played an important role in regulating the mesoderm induction [100]. Therefore, it is not clear if miR-290 has an inhibitory effect on the mesoderm differentiation. Other miRNAs have been shown to have an effect in mesoderm differentiation in zebrafish, such as miR-15 and miR-16 [100], which were also expressed in mouse preimplantation embryos [50].

Mainly, the same miRNAs are expressed during the cleavage divisions of the embryo in mouse and bovine. However, their expression levels often vary during these stages. In murine embryos, the level of miRNA expression is reduced by as much as 60% between one- and two-cell stages. At the end of four-cell stage, mouse embryos have approximately twice as much miRNA compared to the two-cell stage embryo. This implies that the maternally inherited miRNAs degrade at this stage and the EGA starts between the one-cell and four-cell stages [50]. Even though the synthesis and degradation of miRNAs coexists during the preimplantation embryo development in mice, the overall miRNA expression increased towards the blastocyst stage [101].

More than 700 miRNAs have been identified in humans [87, 95, 96, 102]. The level of expression for the majority of these miRNAs stayed the same between the oocyte and the blastocyst stage [87]. More than 50% of the miRNAs expressed in human oocytes and blastocysts were shown to be involved in tumourigenesis, that is, let-7 family, miR-19a, miR-21 and miR-34 [103–109].

4. Gene expression and long noncoding RNAs

In the last few years, in addition to short noncoding RNAs, the lncRNA have gained importance in their roles to affect gene expression. The mammalian genomes consist of long intergenic noncoding RNAs (lincRNAs) that have been suggested to take a role in the regulation of pluripotency during preimplantation embryo development [110]. Human pluripotency transcripts 2, 3 and 5 (HPAT2, HPAT3 and HPAT5) were reported to adjust the pluripotency and ICM formation in preimplantation embryos. Furthermore, HPAT5 was shown to interact with let-7 family of miRNAs [110].

Implantation of embryos involves complex mechanisms and many different genetic and physiological factors are involved during the process. Developing preimplantation embryo must have a good coordinated interaction with the maternal uterine endometrium. LncRNAs were shown to be differentially expressed in endometrial tissues obtained from pigs with pregnancy and non-pregnancy with two lncRNAs, TCONS_01729386 and TCONS_01325501, with potential roles in implantation [111].

5. Gene expression and assisted reproductive technologies

In Western world, approximately 1% of children are born with assisted reproductive technology (ART) treatments. The infertile couples have the best possibility to conceive a child with these treatments. Although these techniques have been considered to be safe in terms of foetal and post-natal development [112, 113], there is an increased risk for morbidities, especially imprinting disorders [114]. Furthermore, the global gene expression profiles vary due to *in vitro* culture of zygotes [115, 116] and *in vitro* fertilisation processes [117]. Following *in vitro* culture, apoptotic and morphogenetic pathways have shown to be altered [118].

Intra-cytoplasmic sperm injection (ICSI), one of the widely used ART techniques, provides infertile couples with sperm motility problems a great chance to have a baby. ICSI is a unique process in which the sperm is injected into the ooplasm [119]. However, ICSI bypasses a number of physiological processes that would normally take place. These embryos derived from ICSI were shown to be cleaved at a slower rate. Furthermore, a reduced number of embryos become hatched with a fewer number of cells and the calcium oscillations are shorter with different patterns [120]. Mice embryos generated by ICSI were shown to be obese and have anomalies of the organs [121].

6. Conclusion

Normal development of preimplantation embryos involves complex mechanisms. For a normal developing embryo, the expression of both maternal and paternal genes is required. Several factors are involved in the regulation of parental genes in preimplantation embryos. Epigenetic modifications are one of the most important factors that are involved in the regulation of gene expression during preimplantation embryos. Extensive research studies have been performed throughout the years to establish the methylation profiles of the mammalian gametes and embryos. In the more recent years, the importance of noncoding RNAs in the regulation of genes has become clear. A handful of studies have been performed to analyse the expression of microRNAs, which have been shown to regulate mRNAs that encode up to 30% human protein-coding genes. The expression of miRNAs has been observed in mouse, bovine and human gametes and embryos. Furthermore, in the last couple of years, expression of long noncoding RNAs and their roles in embryonic development and implantation have been investigated. The extensive research studies have provided crucial understanding of the development of

http://dx.doi.org/10.5772/67851

preimplantation embryos and the regulation of gene expression, and with the advancing technologies more molecular studies will help to comprehend the mechanisms better.

Author details

Pinar Tulay

Address all correspondence to: pinar.tulay@neu.edu.tr

Department of Medical Genetics, Faculty of Medicine, Near East University, Nicosia, North Cyprus

References

[1] Jaroudi, S. and SenGupta, S., DNA repair in mammalian embryos. Mutat Res, 2007. **635**(1): pp. 53-77.

[2] William, L., Human Embryology. Churchill Livingstone New York. Vol. 2nd edition. 1997.

[3] Schultz, R.M., The molecular foundations of the maternal to zygotic transition in the preimplantation embryo. Hum Reprod Update, 2002. **8**(4): pp. 323-31.

[4] Moore, K., Persaud, T.V.N., The Developing Human. 6th ed. Philadelphia:Saunders Company;1998.

[5] Telford, N.A., Watson, A.J., and Schultz, G.A., Transition from maternal to embryonic control in early mammalian development: a comparison of several species. Mol Reprod Dev, 1990. **26**(1): pp. 90-100.

[6] Bell, C.E., Calder, M.D., and Watson, A.J., Genomic RNA profiling and the programme controlling preimplantation mammalian development. Mol Hum Reprod, 2008. **14**(12): pp. 691-701.

[7] McClay, D.W. and Clarke, H.J., Remodelling the paternal chromatin at fertilisation in mammals. Reproduction, 2003. **125**(5): pp. 625-33.

[8] Tamaru, H. and Selker, E.U., A histone H3 methyltransferase controls DNA methylation in Neurospora crassa. Nature, 2001. **414**(6861): pp. 277-83.

[9] Jackson, J.P., et al., Control of CpNpG DNA methylation by the KRYPTONITE histone H3 methyltransferase. Nature, 2002. **416**(6880): pp. 556-60.

[10] Fuks, F., et al., The methyl-CpG-binding protein MeCP2 links DNA methylation to histone methylation. J Biol Chem, 2003. **278**(6): pp. 4035-40.

[11] Morgan, H.D., et al., Epigenetic reprogramming in mammals. Hum Mol Genet, 2005. **14 Spec No 1**: pp. R47-58.

[12] Zhu, B., et al., 5-Methylcytosine DNA glycosylase activity is also present in the human MBD4 (G/T mismatch glycosylase) and in a related avian sequence. Nucleic Acids Res, 2000. **28**(21): pp. 4157-65.

[13] Hardeland, U., et al., The versatile thymine DNA-glycosylase: a comparative characterization of the human, Drosophila and fission yeast orthologs. Nucleic Acids Res, 2003. **31**(9): pp. 2261-71.

[14] Dean, W., Lucifero, D., and Santos, F., DNA methylation in mammalian development and disease. Birth Defects Res C Embryo Today, 2005. **75**(2): pp. 98-111.

[15] Oswald, J., et al., Active demethylation of the paternal genome in the mouse zygote. Curr Biol, 2000. **10**(8): pp. 475-8.

[16] Mayer, W., et al., Demethylation of the zygotic paternal genome. Nature, 2000. **403**. pp. 501-2.

[17] Beaujean, N., et al., Non-conservation of mammalian preimplantation methylation dynamics. Curr Biol, 2004. **14**(7): pp. R266-7.

[18] Reik, W., Dean, W., and Walter, J., Epigenetic reprogramming in mammalian development. Science, 2001. **293**(1089): pp. 1089-93.

[19] Rougier, N., et al., Chromosome methylation patterns during mammalian preimplantation development. Genes Dev, 1998. **12**(14): pp. 2108-13.

[20] Dean, W., et al., Conservation of methylation reprogramming in mammalian development: aberrant reprogramming in cloned embryos. Proc Natl Acad Sci U S A, 2001. **98**(24): pp. 13734-8.

[21] Santos, F. and Dean, W., Epigenetic reprogramming during early development in mammals. Reproduction, 2004. **127**(6): pp. 643-51.

[22] Santos, F., et al., Dynamic reprogramming of DNA methylation in the early mouse embryo. Dev Biol, 2002. **241**(1): pp. 172-82.

[23] Monk, M., Boubelik, M., and Lehnert, S., Temporal and regional changes in DNA methylation in the embryonic, extraembryonic and germ cell lineages during mouse embryo development. Development, 1987. **99**(3): pp. 371-82.

[24] Howlett, S.K. and Reik, W., Methylation levels of maternal and paternal genomes during preimplantation development. Development, 1991. **113**(1): pp. 119-27.

[25] De Vries, W.N., et al., Maternal beta-catenin and E-cadherin in mouse development. Development, 2004. **131**(18): pp. 4435-45.

[26] VB, A., Cell polarity regulator PARD6B is essential for trophectoderm formation in the preimplantation mouse embryo. Biol Reprod, 2010. **83**(3): pp. 347-58.

[27] Ducibella, T., et al., Changes in cell surface and cortical cytoplasmic organization during early embryogenesis in the preimplantation mouse embryo. J Cell Biol., 1977. **74**(1): pp. 153-67.

[28] Kelly, S.J., Studies of the developmental potential of 4- and 8-cell stage mouse blastomeres. J Exp Zool. 1977. **200**(3): pp. 365-76.

[29] Chambers, I., et al., Functional expression cloning of Nanog, a pluripotency sustaining factor in embryonic stem cells. Cell, 2003. **113**(5): pp. 643-55.

[30] Strumpf, D., et al., Cdx2 is required for correct cell fate specification and differentiation of trophectoderm in the mouse blastocyst. Development, 2005. **132**(9): pp. 2093-102.

[31] Nichols, J., et al., Formation of pluripotent stem cells in the mammalian embryo depends on the POU transcription factor Oct4. Cell, 1998. **95**(3): pp. 379-91.

[32] Dietrich, J.E. and Hiiragi, T., Stochastic patterning in the mouse pre-implantation embryo. Development, 2007. **134**(23): pp. 4219-31.

[33] Home, P., et al., Altered subcellular localization of transcription factor TEAD4 regulates first mammalian cell lineage commitment. Proc Natl Acad Sci U S A., 2012. **109**(19): pp. 7362-7.

[34] Paul, S. and Knott, J.G., Epigenetic control of cell fate in mouse blastocysts: the role of covalent histone modifications and chromatin remodeling. Mol Reprod Dev., 2014. **81**(2): pp. 171-82.

[35] Lin, S.C., et al., Klf5 regulates lineage formation in the pre-implantation mouse embryo. Development, 2010 **137**(23): pp. 3953-63.

[36] Davis, T.L., et al., The H19 methylation imprint is erased and re-established differentially on the parental alleles during male germ cell development. Hum Mol Genet, 2000. **9**(19): pp. 2885-94.

[37] Watanabe, D., et al., Stage- and cell-specific expression of Dnmt3a and Dnmt3b during embryogenesis. Mech Dev, 2002. **118**(1-2): pp. 187-90.

[38] Torres-Padilla, M.E., et al., Histone arginine methylation regulates pluripotency in the early mouse embryo. Nature, 2007. **445**(7124): pp. 214-8.

[39] Disteche, C.M., Dosage compensation of the sex chromosomes and autosomes. Semin Cell Dev Biol, 2016. **56**: pp. 9-18.

[40] Namekawa, S.H., et al., Two-step imprinted X inactivation: repeat versus genic silencing in the mouse. Mol Cell Biol, 2010. **30**(13): pp. 3187-205.

[41] Petropoulos, S., et al., Single-cell RNA-Seq reveals lineage and X chromosome dynamics in human preimplantation embryos. Cell, **167**(1): p. 285.

[42] McHugh, C.A., et al., The Xist lncRNA interacts directly with SHARP to silence transcription through HDAC3. Nature, 2015. **521**: pp. 232-236.

[43] Vallot, C., et al., XACT noncoding RNA competes with XIST in the control of X chromosome activity during human early development. Cell Stem Cell. **20**(1): pp. 102-111.

[44] Petropoulos, S., et al., Single-cell RNA-seq reveals lineage and X chromosome dynamics in human preimplantation embryos. Cell. **165**(4): pp. 1012-26.

[45] Amakawa, Y., et al., A new Xist allele driven by a constitutively active promoter is dominated by Xist locus environment and exhibits the parent-of-origin effects. Development, 2015. **142**(24): pp. 4299-308.

[46] Seki, Y., et al., Extensive and orderly reprogramming of genome-wide chromatin modifications associated with specification and early development of germ cells in mice. Dev Biol, 2005. **278**(2): pp. 440-58.

[47] Place, R.F., et al., MicroRNA-373 induces expression of genes with complementary promoter sequences. Proc Natl Acad Sci U S A, 2008. **105**(5): pp. 1608-13.

[48] Plasterk, R.H., Micro RNAs in animal development. Cell, 2006. **124**(5): pp. 877-81.

[49] Tang, F., et al., Maternal microRNAs are essential for mouse zygotic development. Genes Dev, 2007. **21**(6): pp. 644-8.

[50] Lee, R.C., Feinbaum, R.L., and Ambros, V. The C. elegans heterochronic gene lin-4 encodes small RNAs with antisense complementarity to lin-14. Cell. 1993. 75(5): pp. 843-54.

[51] Lee, R.C. and Ambros, V., An extensive class of small RNAs in Caenorhabditis elegans. Science, 2001. **294**(5543): pp. 862-4.

[52] Niwa, R. and Slack, F.J., The evolution of animal microRNA function. Curr Opin Genet Dev, 2007. **17**(2): pp. 145-50.

[53] Tesfaye, D., et al., Identification and expression profiling of microRNAs during bovine oocyte maturation using heterologous approach. Mol Reprod Dev, 2009. **76**(7): pp. 665-77.

[54] Griffiths-Jones, S., et al., miRBase: microRNA sequences, targets and gene nomenclature. Nucleic Acids Res, 2006. **34**(Database issue): pp. D140-4.

[55] Harfe, B.D., et al., The RNaseIII enzyme Dicer is required for morphogenesis but not patterning of the vertebrate limb. Proc Natl Acad Sci U S A, 2005. **102**(31): pp. 10898-903.

[56] Harris, K.S., et al., Dicer function is essential for lung epithelium morphogenesis. Proc Natl Acad Sci U S A, 2006. **103**(7): pp. 2208-13.

[57] Yang, W.J., et al., Dicer is required for embryonic angiogenesis during mouse development. J Biol Chem, 2005. **280**(10): pp. 9330-5.

[58] Muljo, S.A., et al., Aberrant T cell differentiation in the absence of Dicer. J Exp Med, 2005. **202**(2): pp. 261-9.

[59] Ambros, V., The functions of animal microRNAs. Nature, 2004. **431**(7006): pp. 350-5.

[60] Bagga, S., et al., Regulation by let-7 and lin-4 miRNAs results in target mRNA degradation. Cell, 2005. **122**(4): pp. 553-63.

[61] Hayashi, K., et al., MicroRNA biogenesis is required for mouse primordial germ cell development and spermatogenesis. PLoS One, 2008. **3**(3): pp. e1738.

[62] Bartel, D.P., MicroRNAs: genomics, biogenesis, mechanism, and function. Cell, 2004. **116**(2): pp. 281-97.

[63] Bartel, D.P. and Chen, C.Z., Micromanagers of gene expression: the potentially widespread influence of metazoan microRNAs. Nat Rev Genet, 2004. **5**(5): pp. 396-400.

[64] Miranda, K.C., et al., A pattern-based method for the identification of MicroRNA binding sites and their corresponding heteroduplexes. Cell, 2006. **126**(6): pp. 1203-17.

[65] Berezikov, E., et al., Phylogenetic shadowing and computational identification of human microRNA genes. Cell, 2005. **120**(1): pp. 21-4.

[66] Selbach, M., et al., Widespread changes in protein synthesis induced by microRNAs. Nature, 2008. **455**(7209): pp. 58-63.

[67] Baek, D., et al., The impact of microRNAs on protein output. Nature, 2008. **455**(7209): pp. 64-71.

[68] Babiarz, J.E. and Blelloch, R., Small RNAs- their biogenesis, regulation and function in embryonic stem cells. StemBook, 2009. **10.3824**(1.47.1): pp. 1-16.

[69] John, B., et al., Human MicroRNA targets. PLoS Biol, 2004. **2**(11): p. e363.

[70] Filipowicz, W., Bhattacharyya, S.N., and Sonenberg, N., Mechanisms of post-transcriptional regulation by microRNAs: are the answers in sight? Nat Rev Genet, 2008. **9**(2): pp. 102-14.

[71] Berezikov, E., et al., Mammalian mirtron genes. Mol Cell, 2007. **28**(2): pp. 328-36.

[72] Lund, E., et al., Nuclear export of microRNA precursors. Science, 2004. **303**(5654): pp. 95-8.

[73] Yi, R., et al., Exportin-5 mediates the nuclear export of pre-microRNAs and short hairpin RNAs. Genes Dev, 2003. **17**(24): pp. 3011-6.

[74] Schwarz, D.S. and Zamore, P.D., Why do miRNAs live in the miRNP? Genes Dev, 2002. **16**(9): pp. 1025-31.

[75] Giraldez, A.J., et al., MicroRNAs regulate brain morphogenesis in zebrafish. Science, 2005. **308**(5723): pp. 833-8.

[76] Zhao, C., et al., A feedback regulatory loop involving microRNA-9 and nuclear receptor TLX in neural stem cell fate determination. Nat Struct Mol Biol, 2009. **16**(4): pp. 365-71.

[77] Hatfield, S.D., et al., Stem cell division is regulated by the microRNA pathway. Nature, 2005. **435**(7044): pp. 974-8.

[78] Alvarez-Garcia, I. and E.A. Miska, MicroRNA functions in animal development and human disease. Development, 2005. **132**(21): pp. 4653-62.

[79] Barbato, C., et al., Thinking about RNA? MicroRNAs in the brain. Mamm Genome, 2008. **19**(7-8): pp. 541-51.

[80] Davis, T.H., et al., Conditional loss of Dicer disrupts cellular and tissue morphogenesis in the cortex and hippocampus. J Neurosci, 2008. **28**(17): pp. 4322-30.

[81] Giraldez, A.J., et al., Zebrafish MiR-430 promotes deadenylation and clearance of maternal mRNAs. Science, 2006. **312**(5770): pp. 75-9.

[82] Mishima, Y., et al., Differential regulation of germline mRNAs in soma and germ cells by zebrafish miR-430. Curr Biol, 2006. **16**(21): pp. 2135-42.

[83] Zhao, Y., Samal, E., and Srivastava, D., Serum response factor regulates a muscle-specific microRNA that targets Hand2 during cardiogenesis. Nature, 2005. **436**(7048): pp. 214-20.

[84] Harfe, B.D., MicroRNAs in vertebrate development. Curr Opin Genet Dev, 2005. **15**(4): pp. 410-5.

[85] Bernstein, E., et al., Dicer is essential for mouse development. Nat Genet, 2003. **35**(3): pp. 215-7.

[86] Wienholds, E., et al., MicroRNA expression in zebrafish embryonic development. Science, 2005. **309**(5732): pp. 310-1.

[87] McCallie, B., Schoolcraft, W.B., and Katz-Jaffe, M.G., Aberration of blastocyst microRNA expression is associated with human infertility. Fertil Steril, 2009. **93**: pp. 2374-2382.

[88] Maatouk, D.M., et al., Dicer1 is required for differentiation of the mouse male germline. Biol Reprod, 2008. **79**(4): pp. 696-703.

[89] Knight, S.W. and Bass, B.L., A role for the RNase III enzyme DCR-1 in RNA interference and germ line development in Caenorhabditis elegans. Science, 2001. **293**(5538): pp. 2269-71.

[90] Diederichs, S. and Haber, D.A., Dual role for argonautes in microRNA processing and posttranscriptional regulation of microRNA expression. Cell, 2007. **131**(6): pp. 1097-108.

[91] O'Carroll, D., et al., A Slicer-independent role for Argonaute 2 in hematopoiesis and the micro RNA pathway. Genes Dev, 2007. **21**(16): pp. 1999-2004.

[92] Liu, J., et al., Argonaute2 is the catalytic engine of mammalian RNAi. Science, 2004. **305**(5689): pp. 1437-41.

[93] Kurimoto, K., et al., An improved single-cell cDNA amplification method for efficient high-density oligonucleotide microarray analysis. Nucleic Acids Res, 2006. **34**(5): p. e42.

[94] Croce, C.M. and Calin, G.A., miRNAs, cancer, and stem cell division. Cell, 2005. **122**(1): pp. 6-7.

[95] Tulay, P. and Sengupta, S.B., MicroRNA expression and its association with DNA repair in preimplantation embryos. J Reprod Dev., 2016. **62**(3): pp. 225-34.

[96] Tulay P, Naja R.P., Cascales-Roman O., Doshi A., Serhal P., SenGupta S.B., Investigation of microRNA expression and DNA repair gene transcripts in human oocytes and blastocysts. J Assist Reprod Genet, 2015. **32**(12): pp. 1757-64.

[97] Liu, J., et al., MicroRNA-dependent localization of targeted mRNAs to mammalian P-bodies. Nat Cell Biol, 2005. **7**(7): pp. 719-23.

[98] Amanai, M., Brahmajosyula, M., and Perry, A.C., A restricted role for sperm-borne microRNAs in mammalian fertilization. Biol Reprod, 2006. **75**(6): pp. 877-84.

[99] Zovoilis, A., et al., Members of the miR-290 cluster modulate in vitro differentiation of mouse embryonic stem cells. Differentiation, 2009. **78**(2-3): pp. 69-78.

[100] Choi, W.Y., Giraldez, A.J., and Schier, A.F., Target protectors reveal dampening and balancing of Nodal agonist and antagonist by miR-430. Science, 2007. **318**(5848): pp. 271-4.

[101] Yang, Y., et al., Determination of microRNAs in mouse preimplantation embryos by microarray. Dev Dyn, 2008. **237**(9): pp. 2315-27.

[102] Navarro, A. and Monzo, M., MicroRNAs in human embryonic and cancer stem cells. Yonsei Med J, 2010. **51**(5): pp. 622-32.

[103] Chang, T.C., et al., Transactivation of miR-34a by p53 broadly influences gene expression and promotes apoptosis. Mol Cell, 2007. **26**(5): pp. 745-52.

[104] Raver-Shapira, N., et al., Transcriptional activation of miR-34a contributes to p53-mediated apoptosis. Mol Cell, 2007. **26**(5): pp. 731-43.

[105] Paris, R., et al., Multiple p53-independent gene silencing mechanisms define the cellular response to p53 activation. Cell Cycle, 2008. **7**(15): pp. 2427-33.

[106] Lodygin, D., et al., Inactivation of miR-34a by aberrant CpG methylation in multiple types of cancer. Cell Cycle, 2008. **7**(16): pp. 2591-600.

[107] Muller, D.W. and Bosserhoff, A.K., Integrin beta 3 expression is regulated by let-7a miRNA in malignant melanoma. Oncogene, 2008. **27**(52): pp. 6698-706.

[108] Marton, S., et al., Small RNAs analysis in CLL reveals a deregulation of miRNA expression and novel miRNA candidates of putative relevance in CLL pathogenesis. Leukemia, 2008. **22**(2): pp. 330-8.

[109] Hayashita, Y., et al., A polycistronic microRNA cluster, miR-17-92, is overexpressed in human lung cancers and enhances cell proliferation. Cancer Res, 2005. **65**(21): pp. 9628-32.

[110] Durruthy-Durruthy, J., et al., The primate-specific noncoding RNA HPAT5 regulates pluripotency during human preimplantation development and nuclear reprogramming. Nat Genet, 2016. **48**(1): pp. 44-52.

[111] Wang, Y., et al., Analyses of long non-coding RNA and mRNA profiling using RNA sequencing during the pre-implantation phases in pig endometrium. Sci Rep., 2016. **6**: p. 20238.

[112] Anthony, S.B.S., et al., A congenital malformations in 4224 children conceived after IVF. Hum Reprod, 2002. **17**: pp. 2089-95.

[113] DeBaun, M.R., Niemitz, E.L., and Feinberg, A.P., Association of in vitro fertilization with Beckwith-Wiedemann syndrome and epigenetic alterations of LIT1 and H19. Am J Hum Genet 2003. **72**(156-160).

[114] White, C.R., et al., High frequency of imprinted methylation errors in human preimplantation embryos. Sci Rep, 2015. **5**: p. 17311.

[115] Rinaudo, P.F., et al., Effects of oxygen tension on gene expression in preimplantation mouse embryos. Fertil Steril, 2006. **86**(Suppl 4): pp. 1252-65.

[116] Rinaudo, P. and Schultz, R.M., Effects of embryo culture on global pattern of gene expression in preimplantation mouse embryos. Reproduction 2004. **128**: pp. 301-11.

[117] Giritharan, G., et al., Effect of in vitro fertilization on gene expression and development of mouse preimplantation embryos. Reproduction 2007. **134**: pp. 63-72.

[118] Giritharan, G., et al., Effect of ICSI on gene expression and development of mouse preimplantation embryos. Hum Reprod, 2010. **25**(12): pp. 3012-24.

[119] Markoulaki, S., et al., Comparison of Ca2+ and CaMKII responses in IVF and ICSI in the mouse. Mol Hum Reprod, 2007. **13**: pp. 265-72.

[120] Kurokawa, M. and Fissore, R.A., ICSI-generated mouse zygotes exhibit altered calcium oscillations, inositol 1,4,5-trisphosphate receptor-1 downregulation, and embryo development. Mol Hum Reprod, 2003. **9**: pp. 523-33.

[121] Fernandez-Gonzalez, R., et al., Long-term effects of mouse intracytoplasmic sperm injection with DNA-fragmented sperm on health and behavior of adult offspring. Biol Reprod, 2008. **78**: pp. 761-72.

Chapter 6

Non-Invasive Assessment of the Embryo Viability via the Analysis of the Culture Media

Gergely Montskó, Zita Zrínyi, Ákos Várnagy,
József Bódis and Gábor L. Kovács

Additional information is available at the end of the chapter

http://dx.doi.org/10.5772/intechopen.69436

Abstract

Infertility in recent years is a growing public health issue throughout the developed world. Assisted reproductive techniques, especially *in vitro* fertilization, have the potential to partially overcome the low natural reproductive ratio. Nowadays, single embryo transfer gains grounds in clinical practice, urging the development of more reliable methods for selecting the best embryo. In the traditional clinical practice, embryos are selected for transfer based on morphological evaluation. *In vitro* culturing of embryos also provides a very important material for further non-invasive evaluation by means of examining a biomarker in the spent culture medium (SEC). Current measure methods concentrate on the metabolomic activity of the developing embryos none compounds. These studies are mainly utilizing the tools of modern analytics and proteomics. In a paper published by Montskó et al. in 2015, the alpha-1 chain of the human haptoglobin molecule was described as a quantitative biomarker of embryo viability. In a series of retrospective, blind experiments achieved more than 50% success rate. This chapter summarizes the currently available metabolomic and proteomic approaches as the non-invasive molecular assessment of embryo viability.

Keywords: *in vitro* fertilization, embryo viability, non-invasive analysis, proteomics, mass spectrometry, haptoglobin alpha-1 chain

1. Introduction

Nowadays, infertility is a major public health issue affecting couples in the developed world. With the widespread use of assisted reproductive techniques (ARTs), especially *in vitro* fertilization (IVF), there are more and more pregnancies conceived. Currently, approximately 3–4% of all deliveries are IVF pregnancy and this number continues increasing. Availability of ART is a very relevant topic. The cultural and legal conditions, insurance/public funding systems and structure of data collection can influence not only the amount of treatment cycles per inhabitant but also success rates. The Assisted Reproductive Technology National Summary Report of the USA showed a total of 142.000 IVF cycles in 2007 [1], while the most current results in 2014 was 208.604 cycles [2]. The type of ART cycle applied (non-donor or donor egg cycle) is highly varied based on the woman's age. The women younger than 35 years of age often used their own eggs (non-donor) in the majority of cases and just about 4% used donor eggs. However, 38% of women aged 43–44 and 73% of women older than 44 needed to use donor eggs [2]. Similar to the USA, the numbers of ART cycles in Europe show a growing tendency. In 2007, the reported number [3] of treatment cycles was 493.134, while the latest available report describes 640.144 cycles in 2012 [4]. Among the 452.578 fresh cycles reported in 2012, the fraction of IVF and intracytoplasmic sperm injection (ICSI) was 139.978 (31%) and 312.600 (69%), respectively [4]. Despite evolving microsurgical technologies—such as ICSI and some new embryo culturing materials—the rate of successful delivery is far below expectations. In the European IVF monitoring report published in 2016 [4], this rate was 27.8-33.8% depending on the technique of the cycles.

Successful implantation is a complex and bilateral process that requires the selection of a viable embryo and the effective interaction with a receptive endometrium. It is highly unlikely, however, that for the low delivery rate following IVF only maternal reasons would be responsible. In Europe, the total proportion of single embryo transfers (SETs) was 30%. Double embryo transfers occurred in 55% of the cycles, triple embryo transfers were reported in 13% and four or more embryos were transferred in 1% of the cycles. The highest proportions of SETs in 2012 were found in Sweden (76.3%), Finland (75.0%), Norway (60.8%), Belgium (51.1%), Iceland (49.4%), the Czech Republic (47.4%), Austria (46.5%) and Denmark (46.4%) [4]. Nowadays, SET gains grounds in clinical practice. The adoption of an elective SET policy is spreading, urging the development of a reliable method for selecting the most viable embryo, that is, the embryo with the best implantation potential. In the traditional clinical practice of ART, embryos are selected for transfer based on non-invasive morphological evaluation. Several new morphological parameters such as the cleavage rate, blastomere shape and symmetry, and the presence of an adequate trophectoderm layer (TL) or an inner cell mass (ICM) are considered as indicators of implantation potency.

2. Embryo morphology

The most obvious approach for the viability assessment of *in vitro* fertilized embryos is the visual inspection using microscopy. The main reason is the use of any invasive technique such as genetic screening following on-cell embryo biopsy may raise a series of ethical questions. One must not forget that any impact, which affects the embryo during the first days of development, might have undesired late consequences. The choice of morphological parameter depends partly on the time spent after fertilization.

On the first day of development, the morphology of the two pronuclei (the interphase zygotic nuclei) can be graded at 1-cell stage zygotes. Zygote has two pronuclei as the female from the oocyte and the male one from the spermium. Until the end of the interphase of the first embryonic cell cycle, the two pronuclei remain separated. Though on the first day of *in vitro* embryonic development, nucleoli screening is reported to be predictive of pregnancy rate, there are still some disagreements about the usefulness of this morphological marker [5].

The time point of the breakdown of the pronuclear membranes or the time of the first cleavage following fertilization is considered as an indicator of reproductive potential of embryos. Fancsovits et al. reported the relationship of the time point of the pronuclear breakdown with clinical pregnancy and implantation rates. The earliest pronuclear breakdown was at 18 hours after fertilization and the latest time was 31 hours post-insemination. Transferring embryos with the early pronuclear breakdown resulted in a significantly higher clinical pregnancy rate (48.3 vs. 27.3%) and the implantation rates (26.5 vs. 15.1%) [6].

On the second and other later days, the blastomere size, cleavage rate, and pattern of the developing embryo may be evaluated. The best quality embryos supposed to have developed to the four to five blastomere stage on day 2 and have seven or more blastomeres on the third day [5]. Along the number of blastomers, the symmetry of the cleavage is also considered as an indicator of embryo quality. The embryos with symmetric cleavage patterns have a tendency for significantly higher implantation than asymmetric blastomeric shape. Thus, the acceptable cleavage pattern can also be a predictor of implantation outcome [7].

Another important morphological parameter is the grade of fragmentation at the early embryonic development. Cytoplasmic fragments can be found in any human embryo irrespective whether they were fertilized *in vitro* or *in vivo*. The amounts of fragments vary highly, ranging from a few small fragments to a notably high extent of fragmentation involving even blastomere number loss in early cleavage stage embryos. The degree of fragmentation is widely used as an indicator of embryo quality and a predictor of implantation potential. Extensive fragmentation is commonly associated with reduced blastocyst formation and implantation potential. If the degree of fragmentation is below 15%, it seems no effect on blastocyst formation, but more that 15% fragmentation will quickly declines blastocyst formation [8].

The morphological scoring of embryos on 5 and 6 days is also possible by the populations of inner cells (inner cell mass precursors) and outer cells (trophoblast precursors) segregating at about 16-cell stage [9]. An appropriate quality blastocyst has a blastocoel, a trophectoderm layer (TE) and an inner cell mass (ICM). Therefore, the examination of the cell number or the area covered by these cells might be an important factor correlating with embryo viability [5].

It can be seen even on these highlighted examples that there are several options to study the morphology of *in vitro* fertilized embryos and to use these observations to predict implantation potential. It is advised not to select a single parameter, the combination of more than one serves as a better option. The full history of embryo development combining grading of zygotes, cleavage stages and if possible, blastocysts is required to maximize the reliability [5]. Morphological evaluation is an inexpensive method which can be easily implemented in the clinical environment. The biggest drawback of morphological evaluation is that it is a highly subjective method. Therefore, there was a need to form a consensus on these parameters, namely which morphological markers need to be used, what is the weighing of these parameters in the final score, and a scale on which all individual parameters are graded. An international consensus was created in 2011 by the Alpha Scientists in Reproductive Medicine and the European Society of Human Reproduction and Embryology (ESHRE) Special Interest Group of Embryology, based on several morphology markers in different stages of development. The result of this agreement is known as the Istanbul Consensus scoring system. It was expected that standardization of laboratory practice related to embryo morphology assessment will result in more effective comparisons of treatment outcomes worldwide. The document set by the Alpha Scientists group intended to refer as a global standardized consensus for the accurate description of embryo development [10]. The scoring system is composed of several morphological aspects and also considers time spent after fertilization. Nowadays, the guideline sets here serve as the accepted methodology of viability assessment of *in vitro* fertilized embryos.

3. Analysis of the embryo culture medium

Because of ethical reasons, a huge effort is made to find ways of non-invasive viability assessment. The most obvious approach is to study the metabolomic activity of the embryo through the analysis of secreted compounds or by studying the alterations made by the embryo within the culture medium. Due to the importance of the surrounding environment of the embryo and the goal of single embryo transfer concept, and the maintenance of acceptable pregnancy rates, selecting the most optimal culture medium is a crucial point.

First human embryos were cultured in simple salt solutions or in more complex media originally designed for tissue culturing. These early media consisted of physiological salt solutions with added glucose, pyruvate and lactate, and was also supplemented with the patient's serum. Later, it was also revealed that the addition of amino acids to the culture medium increases reproductive potential. Research papers described in both animal and human models that the introduction of amino acids has a positive effect on embryo development and increases viability [11].

Using the experiences published in the literature, several clinics started to develop 'in-house' embryo culturing media, but this way the standardization of culturing circumstances is not an easy task [11]. Therefore, shortly, commercially produced media specifically designed for use in clinical IVF applications was developed satisfying the growing needs. These media are aseptically produced in a specialized factory under standardized conditions, regulations and quality control, and therefore an attractive alternative of 'in-house' embryo culturing media. Nowadays, two types of media exist: sequential culture systems and monoculture systems. Monoculture systems use a single medium composition to support zygote development to the blastocyst stage. The limitation of monoculture systems is that they do not adapt to the altering biochemical needs of the embryo during its development. A medium composition suitable for early cleavage state embryos might not be optimal for the blastocyst stage embryos. Therefore, the majority of IVF clinics use sequential culture systems. It has been determined that conditions that support blastocyst development might inhibit the development of early cleavage stage embryos. If the practice of the clinic covers blastocyst transfer, the sequential medium is the best choice [11].

A very important additive of any type of embryo culturing medium is human serum albumin, which is the most abundant soluble protein constituent of blood described with several physiological roles. In culture medium, albumin serves as pH buffer, an osmotic regulator, membrane stabilizator, a surfactant and a scavenger of metals or toxic substances. Earlier, albumin supplementation was done using human or maternal serum but it has now shifted towards the use of purified albumin products, mainly because of the risk of transferring infectious diseases. With the use of purified albumin products this risk can be eliminated. However, the batch-to-batch stability of different lots of albumin products is sometimes questionable. The use of recombinant albumin might solve all the issues discussed above, but their use is not as widespread as the use of purified albumin products [12].

When dealing with purified albumin products, one must consider that these products are not a 100% pure. In Dyrlund et al.'s recent study [13], 110 proteins other than albumin were identified in commercially available unconditioned culture media supplemented with purified human serum albumin products. Probably it is not an issue in clinical practice since these products have been proven themselves for decades. However, if we use the culture medium as a material for research purpose, it is a very important question.

The measurement of the spent culture medium (SEC) may be served as an exceptional non-invasive alternative in the search of markers of embryo viability. In SEC, the interesting compounds can be divided into two major groups. One consists of compounds present in the unconditioned medium and these compounds may be quantitatively altered by the developing embryo (e.g. nutrients or peptide/protein compounds) [14]. The other group contains embryo-related molecules (e.g. proteins and metabolic end products) secreted by the embryo into the surrounding medium. In order to analyse the secretome of the developing embryo, especially the proteome, it has to be cleared which identified protein originates from the embryo and which was present (or altered in concentration) in the unconditioned medium.

4. Metabolomic studies

The current goal of IVF is to reduce the number of transferred embryos in a single cycle, preferably to only one. Therefore, there is an increasing need for new markers of viability. Numerous factors have been identified as suitable markers of implantation potential, started by the measurement of glucose uptake rate or the determination of pyruvate concentration in the culture medium. Papers reporting such applications in mouse and human models [15, 16] described that blastocysts implanted and developed properly after transferring to the uterus had a significantly higher rate of glucose consumption *in vitro* than those that failed to implant. During the *in vitro* development of human embryos, pyruvate and glucose uptakes were found to be significantly higher by embryos forming normal blastocysts than embryos failing to develop properly. In the first group, an average 22.1 pmol per embryo per hour glucose uptake was recorded, while in the latter group this was only 10.2 pmol per embryo per hour. Comparison of glucose uptakes with morphological embryo grading revealed that the highest glucose uptake was seen in blastocysts of highest grade. Among blastocysts of the same grade from the same patient, there was a notable spread of glucose uptake, indicating that glucose consumption during *in vitro* development may report additional information on embryo viability. It is also described that the measurement of glucose in the medium is more important than that of pyruvate since pyruvate uptakes were similar irrespective of blastocyst grade.

Another option is the examination of amino acid turnover during the early embryonic development by analysing quantitative changes in the amino acid profile of the medium. Amino acids have numerous biological functions during the early period of embryo development. Houghton et al. [17] quantitatively analysed amino acid turnover using high-performance liquid chromatography of individual human embryos. Quantitatively different patterns of amino acid utilization were found between embryos that went on to form a blastocyst and those that failed to develop to blastocyst stage. In the group of normally developing embryos, an increased consumption of leucine from the culture medium was determined. It was also found that the profiles of alanine, arginine, glutamine, methionine, and asparagine predicted developmental potential significantly. Brison et al. [18] revealed alterations in the amino acid concentration of the medium of human zygotes cultured to the 2-cell stage. The turnover of three amino acids, that is, asparagine, glycine, and leucine, was found to be significantly associated with clinical pregnancy and live birth.

Not only selected metabolomic compounds can be examined, but also the analysis of the total metabolome is possible. This area of metabolomic experiments examines the overall metabolic content of the surrounding medium, rather than measuring known nutrients or metabolites. Using analytical techniques such as Raman or near-infrared (NIR) spectroscopy, it is possible to obtain the whole spectral profile of the culture medium surrounding the embryo. It has to be highlighted that it is not possible to identify specific components, it is only possible to detect specific changes to the obtained spectrum. The potential advantage of this approach is an overall analysis for the culture environment [19]. The concept is that after performing spectroscopy at multiple wavelengths in the medium samples of embryos with different implantation outcome, spectral alterations are searched for. These differences are calculated into viability scores or indexes using mathematical algorithms. The observed alterations in the spectra are due to differences in the amount of chemical groups which is a consequence of the metabolic activity of the embryo. The methodology cannot identify the compounds responsible for the spectral differences but indirectly reports information on the metabolomic activity of the developing embryo. For example, if spectral signatures from the near-infrared show differences through the 750–950-nm spectral region, it reports a change in the relative amounts of –OH, –CH and –NH groups [20]. Both Raman and NIR spectroscopic analyses of spent culture media of embryos with known implantation potential demonstrated significantly higher viability indices for embryos representing transfers resulting in clinical pregnancy. When embryos with similar morphology were examined using infrared spectroscopy, viability scores varied remarkably indicating that the analysis of the total metabolome also reports additional information on embryo viability [19]. When calculated viability scores were compared with live birth rates, it was found that embryos having viability scores <0.45 resulted in 19.4% live birth rate, while embryos having viability scores >0.578 resulted in 46.9% live birth rate. This is a very important observation because it clearly indicates that non-invasive metabolomic analysis of the medium of *in vitro* fertilized embryos has its place in the process of viability assessment. Probably a new and additional method cannot replace the existing methodology. However, it can add some new information by identifying markers of low implantation potential unnoticed by the morphological evaluation.

5. Proteomic studies

It is hypothesized that secretory compounds found in the culture medium might provide a characteristic molecular fingerprint. This pattern informs us about embryo growth, developmental competences, and implantation potential. With the emerging of sensitive and specific new analytical techniques, it is possible to carry out a comprehensive analyses of the surrounding environment of pre-implantation embryos [21]. These molecular profiles are supposed to utilize with high accuracy the differentiation of viable and non-viable embryos [22]. The identification of new biomarkers of the embryonic secretome can result in significant improvements in the efficiency of IVF cycles, increasing pregnancy rate per transfer and decreasing the costs of the procedure. There is also a more subjective aspect of more reliable viability assessment: the reduction of the patient's emotional stress [23]. Biological functions are often regulated or carried out by proteins, therefore to understand how a cell or in this case a small population of cells function can be crucial. The analysis of the proteome reports us how the embryo responds to external and also internal conditions. The analysis of the embryonic protein production into the surrounding medium provides a new, molecular perspective of the biochemical pathways activated during the early embryonic development [21].

The proteomic analysis of the embryonic secretome covers the use of the latest analytical tools, very often mass spectrometry (MS) or liquid chromatography-coupled mass spectrometry (LC-MS). MS is probably the most promising technique to study the embryonic secretome. The standard proteomic approach involves separation of intact proteins using 2D gel electrophoresis followed by immediate MS analysis or more likely by digestion and the analysis of the resulting peptide profile. The LC-MS analysis of tryptic digests of control and conditioned embryo culture media, characterization of embryo-related peptides and proteins is now also possible. More recent advances like involving nano-ultra-high pressure chromatography (nano-UPLC) and label-free quantification with mass spectrometry allows the use of minimal amounts of sample and the efficient identification of numerous peptides and proteins in a single analytical run [24]. Matrix-assisted laser-desorption ionization-time-of-flight mass spectrometry (MALDI-TOF) and surface-enhanced laser-desorption ionization-time-of-flight mass spectrometry (SELDI-TOF) are also used to detect different proteins in embryo culture media. SELDI-TOF is a highly sensitive and more importantly a high-throughput method for proteomic analysis, especially for proteins having low molecular weight [21].

Candidates of markers of viability secreted by the embryo cover a broad range of molecules. Sher et al. [25] used the soluble human leukocyte antigen G (sHLA-G) as a predictor of implantation and pregnancy rate. sHLA-G was quantified using an immunoassay and two groups were made according to the quantitative results. Embryos producing sHLA-G above the geometric mean were considered as sHLA-G+ while the ones producing the antigen below the geometric mean were considered as sHLA-G−. In the previous group, significantly higher pregnancy and implantation rates were observed. In the sHLA-G+ group, the pregnancy and implantation rates were 75 and 44%, compared to 23 and 14% of the sHLA-G− group, respectively.

The role of apolipoprotein A1 was also described in Ref. [26] after identification by gel electrophoresis followed by MALDI-TOF MS. Quantification was also performed by ELISA and by quantitative reverse transcriptase polymerase chain reaction of mRNA of apolipoprotein A1. It was found that the level of apolipoprotein A1 correlates with blastocyst grade, but it does not correlate with implantation and pregnancy rates. Contradictory to those findings, Nyalwidhe et al. [22] used MS, Western-blot, and ELISA to identify 14 differentially regulated peptides that were then used to generate genetic algorithms being able to identify embryo transfer cycles resulting in pregnancy and cycles with failed implantation. These genetic algorithms were able to recognize with 71–84% accuracy embryo transfer cycles, which resulted in pregnancy. Several of the 14 peptides were identified as fragments of apolipoprotein A-1, showing reduced expression in media samples representing transfer cycles resulting in viable pregnancies. McReynolds et al. reported an interesting approach based on proteomic analysis [27]. Potential biomarker candidates were selected using an Linear Trap Quadropole-Fourier Transform (LTQ-FT) ultra hybrid mass spectrometer operated in tandem mass spectrometric (MS/MS) mode. Using this proteomic platform, we identified lipocalin-1 to be associated with chromosome aneuploidy. The concentration of lipocalin-1 was determined using a commercially available lipocalin-1 ELISA kit. A clear discrimination of euploid and aneuploid embryos may be determined based on change of lipocalin-1 concentration in micro-drops of culture media. The lipocalin-1 concentration from aneuploid blastocysts showed more significant increase than euploid blastocysts. Pooled micro-drops of euploid embryos contained 3–4 ng/ml of lipocalin-1, while aneuploid embryos contained this compound in a concentration of 6–7 ng/ml. When analysing individual micro-drops of euploid and aneuploid embryos in the spent culture media samples, the results were 4–5 vs. 5–6 ng/ml of lipocalin-1, respectively.

These examples clearly indicate that the non-invasive proteomic analysis of spent culture medium samples has a great potential to determine embryo developmental potency. Thus, this method can be integrated to the existing viability assessing concepts.

6. Viability assessment using quantitative determination of the haptoglobin alpha-1 chain

By LC-MS analysis of spent culture medium samples incubated for 3 days, four different polypeptides were detected and the mass spectra revealed that the monoisotopic masses of the four molecules were 4787.4, 4464.6, 4622.4, and 9186.5 Da, respectively. These numbers showed quantitative difference between the viable (successful pregnancy) and the non-viable (no pregnancy) embryo groups [28]. As the result of various proteomic and statistical considerations, the number of biomarker candidates was reduced to a 9186.5 Da polypeptide. The respective mass spectrum is depicted in **Figure 1**.

Only this compound differed significantly in quantity between the viable and non-viable embryo groups ($p = 0.005$). Proteomic identification was carried out after digestion of the respective chromatographic fraction. By database search using MS data and manual investigation of

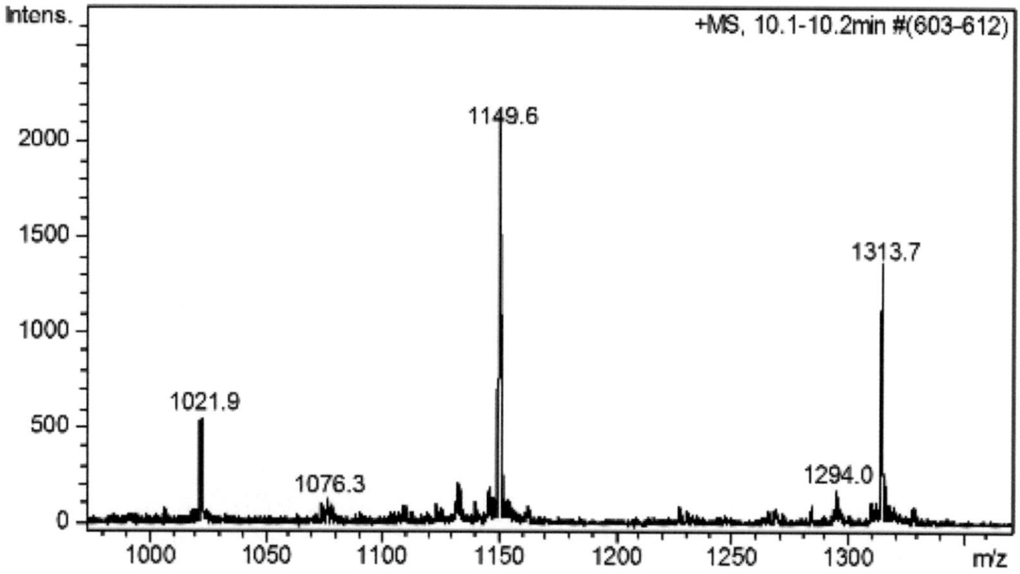

Figure 1. Mass spectrum of the haptoglobin alpha-1 fragment. The horizontal axis represents the measured mass to charge ratio values, displayed as m/z. Absolute peak intensity is shown on the vertical axis. The most intensive peak at m/z 1149.6 corresponds to the [M+8H]8+ ion of the molecule. The peaks at m/z 1021.9 and m/z 1313.7 represent the [M + 9H]9+ and [M + 7H]7+ molecular ions, respectively.

sequence annotations of entries, the protein was identified as the alpha-1 chain of human haptoglobin. The alpha-1 form of this subunit has a monoisotopic mass of 9186.4 Da. All enzymatic fragments identified by tandem mass spectrometry correspond to this region of the haptoglobin precursor protein.

In a set of blind and retrospective experiments including 161 haptoglobin alpha-1 chain measurements, 62 samples were found to be biochemically non-viable and 99 samples were biochemically viable. The biochemically non-viable 62 embryos did not result in any successful baby delivery, while in the biochemically viable group showed 55% pregnancy rate (**Figure 2**). This result revealed a significant difference between viable and non-viable embryo groups ($p < 0.001$) on the basis of the amount of the alpha-1 chain. Moreover, we have found a significant correlation ($p < 0.001$) between the amount of the peptide fragment and the pregnancy outcome.

The probable source of human haptoglobin in the unconditioned medium is the protein contamination of various purified albumin products. The sources of the haptoglobin alpha-1 chain in the culture medium are due to the reduction of the disulphide bonds connecting the chains of the matured haptoglobin molecule. The explanation for the increased amount of alpha-1 chain in the samples of non-viable embryos might be the fact that abnormally developing or damaged embryos often show the characteristics of apoptosis in a larger extent than normal embryos. Apoptosis later might be followed by secondary necrosis accompanied by increased membrane permeability. We hypothesize that these processes might result in the release of enzymes or other chemical factors from the cells of abnormally developing embryos altering the chemical environment in the medium.

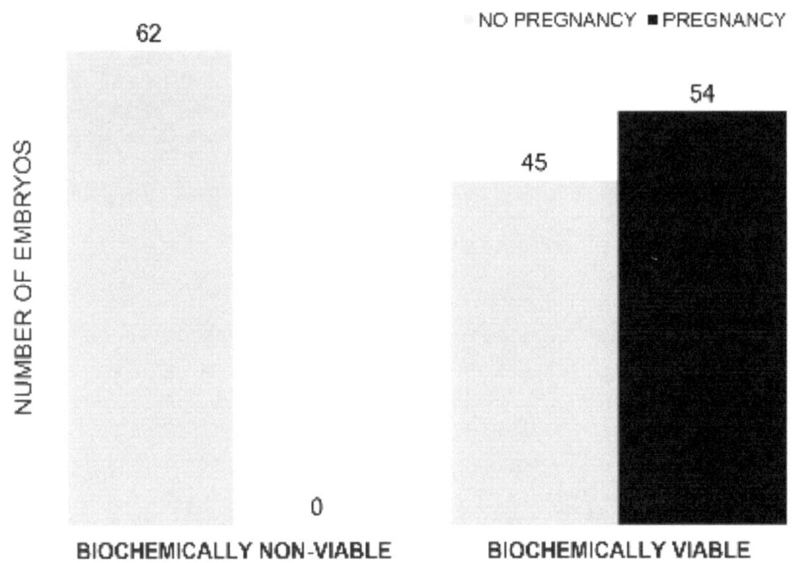

Figure 2. Results of the blinded analysis of embryo culture medium after 3 days of incubation (n = 161). In the group assessed as biochemically non-viable, no pregnancy was found. Embryos assessed as biochemically viable, showed an 55% pregnancy rate.

7. Apoptosis during early embryonic development

Programmed cell death (PCD)—also called apoptosis—is a well-known biological phenomenon. It is characterized by cell membrane blebbing, chromatin condensation and DNA fragmentation, involving several membrane receptors and the activation of signal transduction pathways. Classic signs of apoptosis are cell shrinkage, nuclear condensation, and the formation of vesicles called 'apoptotic bodies'. The most significant biochemical event associated with apoptosis is DNA fragmentation producing a specific gel electrophoresis picture called the DNA ladder. Apoptosis *in vivo* occurs in every multicellular organism and is an essential biological process [29].

Normal apoptosis in early embryos is crucial for proper development. In blastocysts, for example, both the inner cell mass and the trophectoderm layer undergo apoptosis [29]. Apoptosis during the normal development of the pre-implantation embryos has several functions. It is hypothesized that the cell number in the inner mass of the blastocyst follows an equilibrium and apoptosis helps to maintain cellular homeostasis. The other possible reason for PCD during early development is the elimination of cells with an abnormally altered genetic constitution or cells having other abnormalities or inadequate developmental potential. For example, within the inner cell mass, the appearance of aneuploid cells is well known. The markers of apoptosis are also considered as additional features for oocyte and embryo quality assessment. Arrested embryos tend to have a high grade of apoptosis [30].

Apoptotic cells should be normally phagocytosed, however, if it is not possible they may undergo secondary necrosis, which differs from apoptosis by an increase in membrane permeability and excretion of cytosolic structures. These events are observed in a variety of different cell types [31]. The apoptotic program provides two alternative ways of cell elimination. Early surface signals can allow scavenger phagocytes to recognize apoptotic cells and remove them with a 'silent' elimination process. Secondary necrosis occurs in the absence of scavenger cells leading to a final autolytic disintegration. These cells exhibit specific apoptotic signs and also necrotic features, for example, the degradation of the cytoplasmic membrane. Secondary necrosis might also occur *in vivo* accompanying several pathological cases when functioning scavenger cells are not available [32]. *In vitro* apoptosis tends to proceed in a similar way involving the activation of hydrolytic enzymes and a damage of the cytoplasmic membrane, resulting in cell disruption. This process occurs if the removal of the apoptotic cells or apoptotic bodies fails. The events described in the process of primary necrosis are operating during secondary necrosis, too. The mechanism of cell death involves proteolysis due to the activity of proteinases causing an additional release of cytosolic compounds [33]. Studies on animal models indicate that *in vitro* culturing increases PCD and that the composition of the medium can affect the incidence of the process. The reason is that the culture medium lacks some crucial maternal 'survival' factors [31]. We hypothesize that during the *in vitro* culturing an increased PCD is observed, resulting in secondary necrosis because of the absence of scavenging cells in the artificial *in vitro* environment. The described phenomenon of haptoglobin cleavage might be a result of factors released from the embryonic cells due to secondary necrosis and increased membrane permeability.

8. Concluding remarks

Our detailed study showed that the alpha-1 chain of the human haptoglobin molecule may be used as a biomarker to distinguish the *in vitro* culture embryo implantation ability, which yet has not been proven earlier by others to be an indicator of embryo viability. The embryos diagnosed as biochemically non-viable did not lead to pregnancy at all. However, the embryos that were classified as biochemically viable showed a 55% pregnancy rate, while the control only showed the 30% pregnancy rate without the measurement of the haptoglobin alpha-1 fragment. The authors think that non-invasive metabolomic and proteomic approaches might have a place in the process of routine IVF but cannot substitute the process of morphological assessment. An ideal practice of IVF might contain a step ruling out the morphologically worst embryos followed by a laboratory measurement of the haptoglobin alpha-1 chain of media of the remaining ones. The main disadvantage of this technique is the application of mass spectrometry in the routine process of IVF, which requires an expensive laboratory background and is usually not available in the reproductive units. The developing field of lab-on-a-chip concept in combination with already existing point-of-care medical instruments can be a possible end point [34].

Acknowledgements

The presented work was supported by Hungarian Scientific Research Fund – OTKA/115394/2015/HU "Early biochemical indicators of embryo viability", EDIOP-2.3.2-15-2016-00021/HU "The use of chip-technology in increasing the effectiveness of human *in vitro* fertilization", EFOP-3.6.1.-16-2016-00004 Comprehensive Development for Implementing Smart Specialization Strategies at the University of Pécs and by the ÚNKP-17-4-III "New National Excellence Program of the Ministry of Human Capacities" grants.

Author details

Gergely Montskó[1,2], Zita Zrínyi[1], Ákos Várnagy[2,3], József Bódis[2,3] and Gábor L. Kovács[1,2,4]*

*Address all correspondence to: kovacs.l.gabor@pte.hu

1 Szentágothai Research Centre, University of Pécs, Pécs, Hungary

2 MTA-PTE Human Reproduction Scientific Research Group, University of Pécs, Pécs, Hungary

3 Department of Obstetrics and Gynecology, University of Pécs, Pécs, Hungary

4 Department of Laboratory Medicine, University of Pécs, Pécs, Hungary

References

[1] Seli E, Sakkas D, Scott R, Kwok SC, Rosendahl SM, Burns DH. Noninvasive metabolomic profiling of embryo culture media using Raman and near-infrared spectroscopy correlates with reproductive potential of embryos in women undergoing in vitro fertilization. Fertility and Sterility. 2007;**88**:1350-1357. DOI :10.1016/j.fertnstert.2007.07.1390

[2] 2014 Assisted Reproductive Technology National Summary Report.[Internet] 2014. Available from: https://www.cdc.gov/art/pdf/2014-report/art-2014-national-summary-report.pdf

[3] de Mouzon J, Goossens V, Bhattacharya S, Castilla JA, Ferraretti AP, Korsak V, Kupka M, Nygren KG, Andersen AN. Assisted reproductive technology in Europe, 2007: Results generated from European registers by ESHRE. Human Reproduction. 2012;**4**:954-966. DOI :10.1093/humrep/des023

[4] European IVF-Monitoring Consortium (EIM) for the European Society of Human Reproduction and Embryology (ESHRE), Calhaz-Jorge C, de Geyter C, Kupka MS, de Mouzon J, Erb K, Mocanu E, Motrenko T, Scaravelli G, Wyns C, Goossens V. Assisted reproductive technology in Europe, 2012: Results generated from European registers by ESHRE. Human Reproduction. 2016;**31**:1638-1652. DOI: 10.1093/humrep/dew151

[5] Ajduk A, Zernicka-Goetz M. Quality control of embryo development. Molecular Aspects of Medicine. 2013;**34**:903-918. DOI: 10.1016/j.mam.2013.03.001

[6] Fancsovits P, Toth L, Takacs ZF, Murber A, Papp Z, Urbancsek J. Early pronuclear breakdown is a good indicator of embryo quality and viability. Fertility and Sterility. 2005;**84**:881-887. DOI:10.1016/j.fertnstert.2005.03.068

[7] Sela R, Samuelov L, Almog B, Schwartz T, Cohen T, Amit A, Azem F, Ben-Yosef D. An embryo cleavage pattern based on the relative blastomere size as a function of cell number for predicting implantation outcome. Fertility and Sterility. 2012;**98**:650-656.e4. DOI: 10.1016/j.fertnstert.2012.05.041

[8] Hardy K, Stark J, Winston RML. Maintenance of the inner cell mass in human blastocysts from fragmented embryos. Biology of Reproduction. 2003;**68**:1165-1169. DOI: 10.1095/biolreprod.102.010090

[9] Boiso I, Veiga A, Edwards RG. Fundamentals of human embryonic growth in vitro and the selection of high-quality embryos for transfer. Reproductive BioMedicine Online. 2002;**5**:328-350

[10] Alpha Scientists in Reproductive Medicine and ESHRE Special Interest Group of Embryology. Istanbul consensus workshop on embryo assessment. Proceedings of an Expert Meeting. Reproductive BioMedicine Online. 2011;**22**:632-646. DOI: 10.1016/j.rbmo.2011.02.001

[11] Lane M, Gardner DK. Embryo culture medium: Which is the best? Best Practice & Research Clinical Obstetrics & Gynaecology. 2007;**21**:83-100. DOI:10.1016/j.bpobgyn.2006.09.009

[12] Blake D, Svalander P, Jin M, Silversand C, Hamberger L. Protein supplementation of human IVF culture media. Journal of Assisted Reproduction and Genetics. 2002;**19**:137-143

[13] Dyrlund TF, Kirkegaard K, Poulsen ET, Sanggaard KW, Hindkjær JJ, Kjems J, Enghild JJ, Ingerslev HJ. Unconditioned commercial embryo culture media contain a large variety of non-declared proteins: A comprehensive proteomics analysis. Human Reproduction. 2014;**29**:2421-30. DOI: 10.1093/humrep/deu220

[14] Rødgaard T, Heegaard PM, Callesen H. Non-invasive assessment of in-vitro embryo quality to improve transfer success. Reproductive BioMedicine Online. 2015;**31**:585-592. DOI: 10.1016/j.rbmo.2015.08.003

[15] Gardner DK, Wale PL. Analysis of metabolism to select viable human embryos for transfer. Fertility and Sterility. 2013;**99**:1062-1072. DOI: 10.1016/j.fertnstert.2012.12.004

[16] Gardner DK, Lane M, Stevens J, Schoolcraft WB. Noninvasive assessment of human embryo nutrient consumption as a measure of developmental potential. Fertility and Sterility. 2001;**76**:1175-1180

[17] Houghton FD, Hawkhead JA, Humpherson PG, Hogg JE, Balen AH, Rutherford AJ, Leese HJ. Non-invasive amino acid turnover predicts human embryo developmental capacity. Human Reproduction. 2002;**17**:999-1005.

[18] Brison DR, Houghton FD, Falconer D, Roberts SA, Hawkhead J, Humpherson PG, Lieberman BA, Leese HJ. Identification of viable embryos in IVF by noninvasive measurement of amino acid turnover. Human Reproduction 2004;**19**:2319-2324. DOI:10.1093/humrep/deh409

[19] Vergouw CG, Botros LL, Judge K, Henson M, Roos P, Kostelijk EH, Schats R, Twisk JW, Hompes PG, Sakkas D, Lambalk CB. Non-invasive viability assessment of day-4 frozen-thawed human embryos using near infrared spectroscopy. Reproductive BioMedicine Online. 2011;**23**:769-776. DOI: 10.1016/j.rbmo.2011.08.015

[20] Seli E, Sakkas D, Scott R, Kwok SC, Rosendahl SM, Burns DH. Noninvasive metabolomic profiling of embryo culture media using Raman and near-infrared spectroscopy correlates with reproductive potential of embryos in women undergoing in vitro fertilization. Fertility and Sterility. 2007;**88**:1350-1357. DOI: 10.1016/j.fertnstert.2007.07.1390

[21] Katz-Jaffe MG, Schoolcraft WB, Gardner DK. Analysis of protein expression (secretome) by human and mouse preimplantation embryos. Fertility and Sterility. 2006;**86**:678-685. DOI:10.1016/j.fertnstert.2006.05.022

[22] Nyalwidhe J, Burch T, Bocca S, Cazares L, Green-Mitchell S, Cooke M, Birdsall P, Basu G, Semmes OJ, Oehninger S. Molecular Human Reproduction. 2013;**19**:250-263. DOI: 10.1093/molehr/gas063

[23] Poli M, Ori A, Child T, Jaroudi S, Spath K, Beck M, Wells D. Characterization and quantification of proteins secreted by single human embryos prior to implantation. EMBO Molecular Medicine. 2015;**7**:1465-1479. DOI: 10.15252/emmm.201505344

[24] Cortezzi SS, Garcia JS, Ferreira CR, Braga DP, Figueira RC, Iaconelli A Jr, Souza GH, Borges E Jr, Eberlin MN. Secretome of the preimplantation human embryo by bottom-up label-free proteomics. Analytical and Bioanalytical Chemistry. 2011;**401**:1331-1339. DOI: 10.1007/s00216-011-5202-1

[25] Sher G, Keskintepe L, Fisch JD, Acacio BA, Ahlering P, Batzofin J, Ginsburg M. Soluble human leukocyte antigen G expression in phase I culture media at 46 hours after fertilization predicts pregnancy and implantation from day 3 embryo transfer. Fertility and Sterility. 2005;**83**:1410-1413. DOI: 10.1016/j.fertnstert.2004.11.061

[26] Mains LM, Christenson L, Yang B, Sparks AE, Mathur S, Van Voorhis BJ. Identification of apolipoprotein A1 in the human embryonic secretome. Fertility and Sterility. 2011;**96**:422-427.e2. DOI: 10.1016/j.fertnstert.2011.05.049

[27] McReynolds S, Vanderlinden L, Stevens J, Hansen K, Schoolcraft WB, Katz-Jaffe MG. Lipocalin-1: A potential marker for noninvasive aneuploidy screening. Fertility and Sterility. 2011;**95**:2631-2633. DOI: 10.1016/j.fertnstert.2011.01.141

[28] Montskó G, Zrínyi Z, Janáky T, Szabó Z, Várnagy Á, Kovács GL, Bódis J. Noninvasive embryo viability assessment by quantitation of human haptoglobin alpha-1 fragment in the in vitro fertilization culture medium: an additional tool to increase success rate. Fertility and Sterility. 2015;**103**:687-693. DOI: 10.1016/j.fertnstert.2014.11.031

[29] Brill A, Torchinsky A, Carp H, Toder V. The role of apoptosis in normal and abnormal embryonic development. Journal of Assisted Reproduction and Genetics. 1999;**16**:512-519

[30] Haouzi D, Hamamah S. Pertinence of apoptosis markers for the improvement of in vitro fertilization (IVF). Current Medical Chemistry. 2009;**16**:1905-1916

[31] Hardy K. Apoptosis in the human embryo. Reviews of Reproduction. 1999;**4**:125-134

[32] Silva MT. Secondary necrosis: the natural outcome of the complete apoptotic program. FEBS Letters. 2010;**584**:4491-4499. DOI: 10.1016/j.febslet.2010.10.046

[33] Silva MT, do Vale A, dos Santos NM. Secondary necrosis in multicellular animals: An outcome of apoptosis with pathogenic implications. Apoptosis. 2008;**13**:463-482. DOI: 10.1007/s10495-008-0187-8

[34] Le Gac S, Nordhoff V. Microfluidics for mammalian embryo culture and selection: Where do we stand now? Molecular Human Reproduction. 2017;**23**:213-226. DOI:10.1093/molehr/gaw061

Section 4

Improving Embryo Cleavage Technology

Chapter 7

Improving ART Pregnancy Rate with Two Kinds of Media and Two Types of Incubators

Bin Wu, Jinzhou Qin, Suzhen Lu, Linda Wu and Timothy J. Gelety

Additional information is available at the end of the chapter

http://dx.doi.org/10.5772/intechopen.70062

Abstract

Culture media and incubators have played a key role in embryo quality. Here, we observed individual patient's embryos to have different response for media and incubators. Patient's 1850 zygotes were divided into two groups randomly and were cultured in Global and in P1 medium. The cleavage rate and embryo quality were recorded. The result showed that the cleavage, top quality embryos on Day 2 and Day 3 were not statistically different between media. However, 45% patient's embryos grew very well in both Global and P1. 22% patient's embryos grew well only in Global but poor quality in P1, while 21% grew well in the Global but poorly in the P1. Only 12% patient embryos did not grow well in both. The pregnant rate was only 40% in P1 or 42.5% in Global (P>0.05). However, when two media were used simultaneously, the pregnant rate increased to 70.1%. Also, two incubators showed significant higher pregnant rate than in single incubator (73.2% vs. 60%, P<0.05). In conclusion, the favorable response of individual patient's embryos to media and incubators suggests that using two media and two incubators for embryo culture could significantly improve embryo quality and pregnant rates.

Keywords: medium, incubator, IVF, pregnancy, outcome

1. Introduction

Assisted reproductive technology (ART) including in vitro fertilization (IVF) and intracytoplasmic sperm injection (ICSI) has now widely been used for the treatment of infertility. The successful application of this technology to human ART is mainly due to embryo culture environment innovation including culture media and incubators. So far, different culture systems have been successfully used for *in vitro* production of human and animal embryos.

Since the first rabbit embryo culture was described in 1912 [1, 2], mouse zygote could be cultured to form blastocyst stage embryos in a complex culture medium [3]. In 1985, an embryo culture medium called human tubal fluid medium (HTF) was first described as designed specifically for human IVF [4]. Since the development of HTF, many modifications and advancements have been made in the recipes for human embryo culture medium.

For many decades, optimization of culture media for the support of human and animal embryos has been a focus of considerable interest [5]. As the further understanding of both the physiological changes in oviduct and uterus and the different metabolic needs of cleavage and blastocyst stage embryos, the many novel embryo culture media are continually developed. Currently, several types of media are available in the market representing different strategies and generally fall into one of the three types: (1) simple salt solutions with added energy substrates, such as KSOM, P1, etc., [6, 7]; (2) complex tissue culture media, such as Ham's F-10 [8]; and (3) sequential media, such as G1/G2, and developed G5 serious media [9]. More recently, sequential culture media have been produced to take into account the changing metabolic needs of the embryo from the cleavage to the blastocyst stage [10, 11]. So far, many commercial embryo culture media are available for human embryo culture and their effect for embryo culture is various [12]. At present, when we search with key words "human embryo culture medium comparison" in google.com, the 53,600 results will occur at 0.6 s. The studies comparing these medium effects on embryonic development have reported contradictory conclusion. Many studies did not find a significant difference or just tiny difference between various culture media [13, 14]. Recently, Mantikou et al. [15] used meta-analysis to evaluate 31 different comparisons for 20 different culture media and did not find what culture medium leads to the best success rates in IVF/ICSI.

We think that significant differences of various media for embryo culture may be difficult to be demonstrated because every commercial company for human embryo culture media must continuously improve the quality of its available culture media. Thus, most of the current commercial culture media may produce satisfied results for human embryo culture. Therefore, the choice of the best culture medium in each laboratory has been attributed to embryologist interesting and specific work conditions.

Also, incubators in the IVF laboratory play a pivotal role in providing a stable and appropriate culture environment required for optimizing embryo development and clinical outcomes. With technological advances, several types of incubators have been applied to human IVF laboratory. Recently, Swain [16] did a comparative analysis of embryo cultural incubators in human IVF laboratories and reviewed some incubator functions and key environmental variables controlled and the technology utilized in various units. This comparison indicates that smaller bench top/top load incubators provide faster recovery of environmental variables, but there is no clear advantage of any particular incubator based on clinical outcomes.

Based on the last decade practice of our IVF center, there was no any difference on embryo culture between Cook Minc incubator and front-door big-box incubator. However, we observed that the same patient's sibling embryos for splitting into two medium cultures often have different development results under the condition of different incubators. Our question is whether patient's embryos have a favorable selection for culture medium or incubator condition? The objective of this study is to determine whether specific differences of patient embryos in response to culture media and incubator are important in the human embryo culture system.

2. Materials and methods

2.1. Culture media

This study mainly used two media for embryo culture: P1 medium is from Irvine Scientific, Inc, CA, and Life-Global medium is from Life Global, LLC, Canada. Two kinds of media added 10% serum substitute supplement (SSS) (Irvine Scientific, Inc, CA) for embryo culture.

2.2. Culture incubators

Forma water-jacketed CO_2 incubator is from Thermal Forma Scientific, Inc, and this incubator is just connected to medical grade CO_2 gas tank and is adjusted to 5% CO_2 for embryo culture. Cook Benchtop Incubator was connected to the certified premixed tri-gas tank which contained 5% O_2, 6% CO_2, and 89% N (**Figure 1**). Although two incubators connected with different CO_2 concentration, their pH tests showed the range from 7.21 to 7.38 and no significant difference was observed between two medium in two types of incubators.

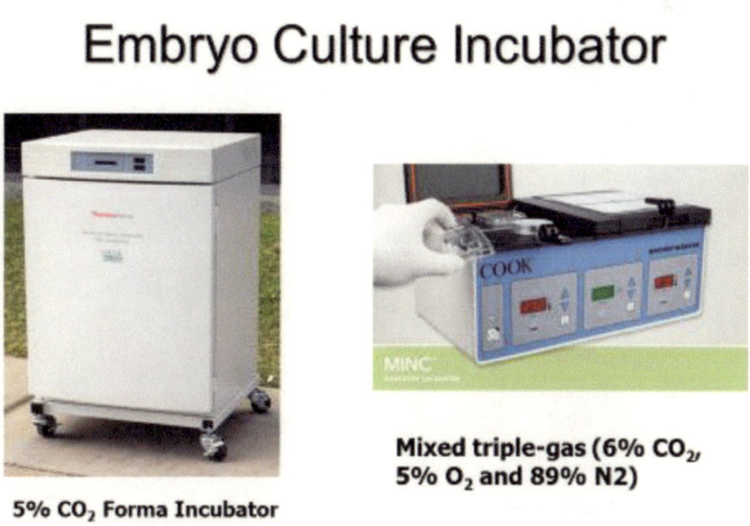

Figure 1. Embryo culture incubators. Two kinds of incubators are shown as big-box incubator (left) and Cook Bench Minc incubator (right).

3. Experiment design

This was a prospective randomized study of infertility couples undergoing assisted reproductive procedures during 2012–2013 at the Arizona Center for Reproductive Endocrinology and Infertility. During this period, all patients (age 25–43) were treated by our standard stimulation protocol (LA/HMG, HCG 10,000 IU/ml) before oocyte retrieval. The retrieval oocytes were cultured in P1 medium (Irvine Scientific, Inc) with 3% human serum albumin (HSA, InVitoCare, Frederick, MD) for 4–6 h at 37°C with 5% CO_2 incubator. Then, oocytes were routinely inseminated in 100 μl of P1 medium microdrops for in vitro fertilization or conducted by intracytoplasmic sperm injection depending on husband sperm quality (approximately 35% of cycles required ICSI). Fertilization was assessed on the following day, 18–20 h after insemination or ICSI. If two distinct pronuclei (2PN) were observed, the fertilization was confirmed. The zygotes per patient were randomly divided into two groups and cultured in either P1 medium or Life-Global medium in petri dishes with each drop of 50 μl culture medium for another 2 days (see experimental design, **Figure 2**).

Each embryo was cultured in an individual microdrop. The status of embryo cleavage and quality were assessed after a further 24 and 48 h of in vitro culture. The embryonic grade was evaluated according to the number and size equality of blastomeres, presence or absence of granularity, and the relative proportion of anucleate fragments by at least two experienced embryologists by 100X magnification on an inverted microscope. Based on our standard criteria, good-quality or top-quality embryos (Grade 5) were defined as regular, spherical blastomeres with less 10% extracellular fragmentations and had 6–10 blastomeres on day 3. Embryos with Grade 1–4 were defined as low quality. On the day of embryo transfer (ET), one

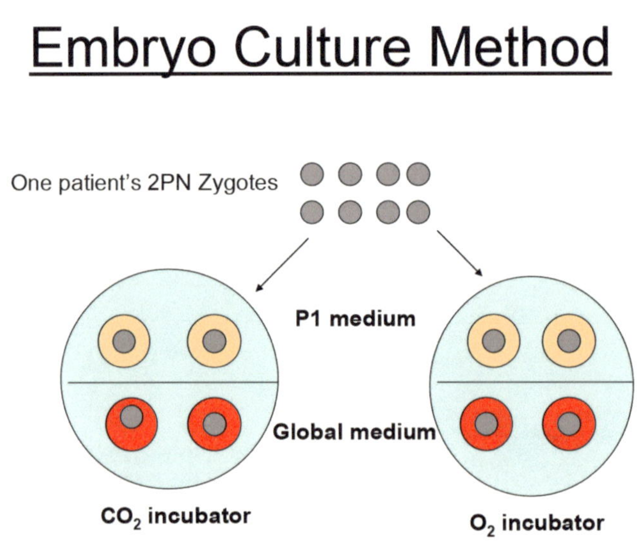

Figure 2. Embryo culture method. A patient sibling fertilized zygotes were randomly divided into two media and two incubators for culture.

to four embryos were selected for abdominal ultrasound-guided transfer to uterus according to patient age and embryo quality. The transferred embryos from each medium or incubator were recorded. The most of, most of the best quality embryos for transfer were selected from two media and two incubators. The remaining embryos, if any, were left in the culture dish to undergo cryopreservation. Clinical pregnancy was diagnosed by the presence of a gestational sac by ultrasound echographic screening approximately 5–6 weeks after the embryo replacement procedure.

Statistical analysis was performed using student *t*-test. Significant statistical difference was considered as $P<0.05$.

4. Results

4.1. New discovery

In 2008–2009, we often observed that the patient's embryos had a different response to each medium. Some patient's embryos favored to grow in the global medium, while some patient's embryos preferred to live in the P1 medium and some embryos grew very well in both global medium and P1 medium, which means that embryos have a favorable selectivity to medium (**Figure 3**).

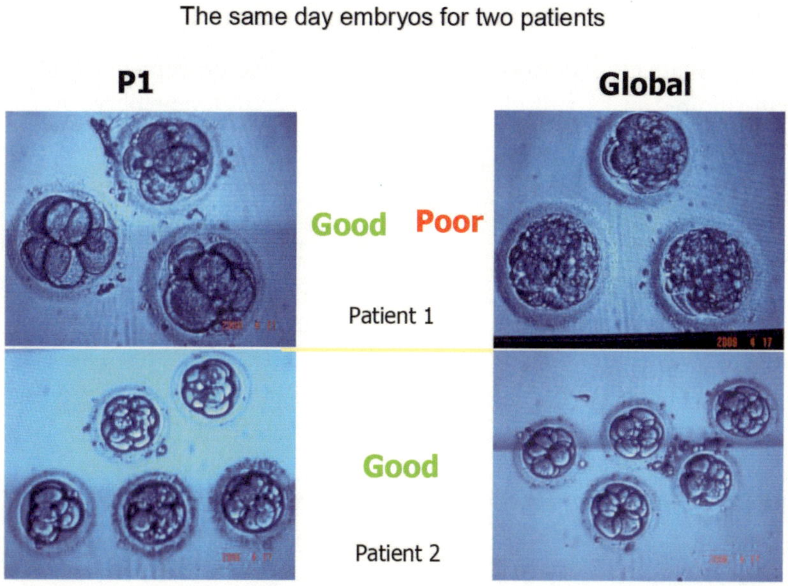

Figure 3. The patient's embryo response to two media. On the same day, two patients' embryos were placed in the two medium culture. Patient 1 embryos grew very well in the P1 medium (left), but they had a lot of fragmentation in global medium (right). However, the 10 embryos of patient 2 grew very well in both media.

4.2. Experimental verification

In order to verify our former observation, two different commercially available media (P1 and Life-Global media) were used in this study. A total of 1850 normal fertilized 2PN zygotes from 220 consecutive patient cycles were studied. The cleavage rate and top-quality embryos on day 2 and day 3 were compared. Results indicated the same zygote cleavage rate for two media, and global medium seemed to yield slightly higher top-quality embryos on day 2 and day 3, but it was not statistically different between two media (*P*>0.05, **Table 1** and **Figure 4**). When patient's sibling embryos were cultured in two different incubators, their cleavage and the top embryo of day 2 and day 3 also did not show any significant difference (*P*>0.05, **Figure 5**).

However, when the patient sibling embryos were cultured in two media, some patient embryos developed very well in the P1 medium, while some patient embryos grew well in global medium. Here, we gave four patient samples to show the responses of patient embryos to two culture media (**Figures 6–9**).

Patient A was 38 years old. Five oocytes were retrieved on September 30, 2013, and four zygotes were individually cultured in P1 and global medium in Forma incubator and Cook Minc incubator, respectively. On day 3, all embryos showed a good quality under the various conditions

Patient B was 23 years old. Thirteen oocytes were retrieved on October 4, 2013, and four zygotes were individually cultured in P1 and global medium in Forma incubator and Cook Minc incubator, respectively. On day 3, all embryos showed a low quality and slow growing under the various conditions.

Patient C was 33 years old. Fourteen oocytes were retrieved on September 30, 2013, and 11 zygotes were cultured in P1 and global microdrop medium (one embryo in each drop) in

Embryo grade	Medium				Incubator			
	Global		P1		Forma		Minc	
	Embryos/total	%	Embryos/total	%	Embryos/total	%	Embryos/total	%
Cleavage	907/930	97.5[a]	808/920	98.7[a]	992/1025	96.8[a]	807/825	97.8[a]
Day 2 top-quality embryos	633/845	74.9[a]	624/836	74.6[a]	730/988	73.9[a]	598/800	74.8[a]
Day 3 top-quality embryos	564/857	65.8[a]	477/768	62.1[a]	573/902	63.3[a]	478/726	65.8[a]

[a]No significant difference between two medium groups (*P*>0.05).

Some patient embryos were not observed on day 2 and were observed on day 3. Day 2 top-quality embryo shows 2–6 cells/Grade 5 and day 3 top-quality embryo shows 5–8 cells/Grade 5.

Table 1. Effect of culture media and incubators on zygote development.

http://dx.doi.org/10.5772/intechopen.70062

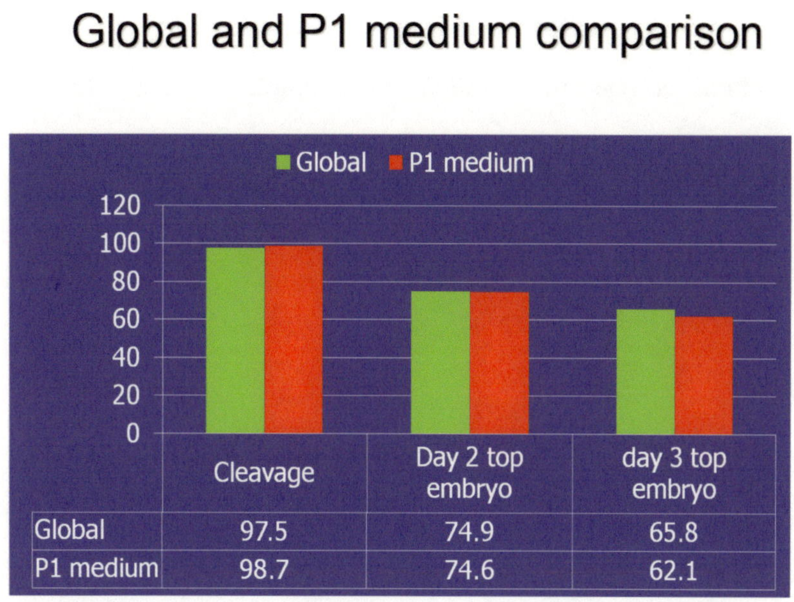

Figure 4. Patient embryos cultured in two medium did not show any significant difference on cleavage, day 2 and day 3 high-quality embryos.

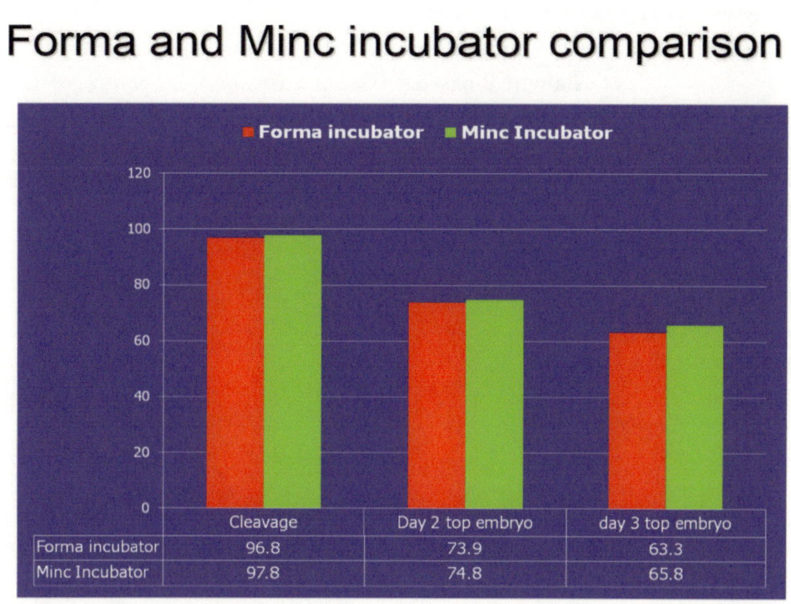

Figure 5. Patient embryos cultured in two different incubators did not show any significant difference on cleavage, day 2 and day 3 high-quality embryos.

Forma incubator and Cook Minc incubator, respectively. On day 3, only three good-quality embryos were obtained in the global medium in the Cook Minc incubator. Other eight embryos showed low quality under other three kinds of condition.

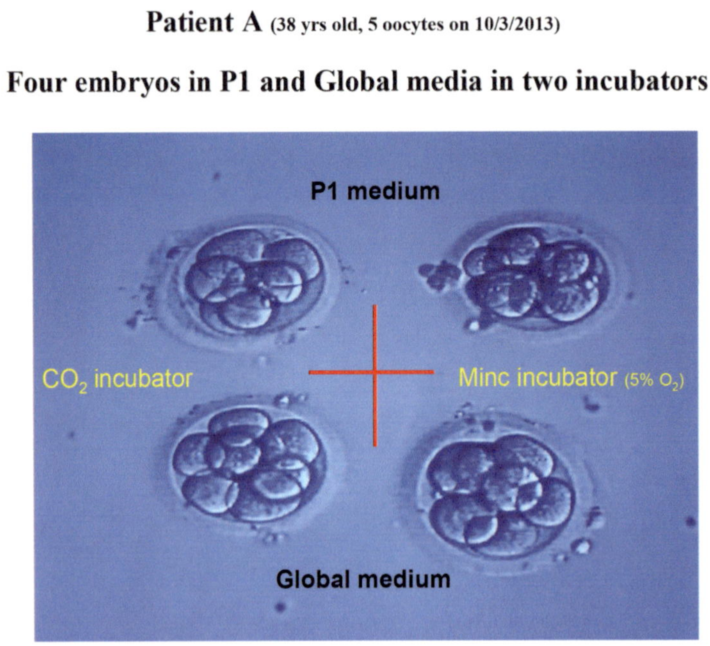

Figure 6. The four embryos of a 38-year-old woman showed very well growing in two media and two incubators. Day 3 embryos were displayed under the same microscope view.

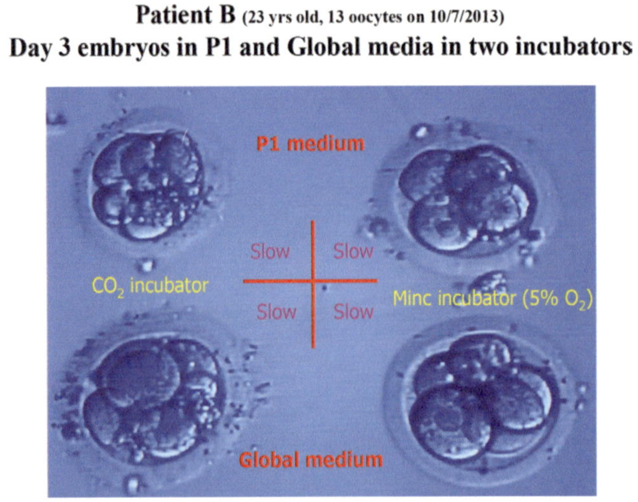

Figure 7. The four embryos of a 23-year-old woman showed very poor growing in two media and two incubators. Day 3 embryos were displayed under the same microscope view.

Patient D was 41 years old. Five oocytes were retrieved on October 4, 2013, and five zygotes were individually cultured in P1 and global medium in Forma incubator and Cook Minc incubator, respectively. On day 3, only one embryo in P1 medium with Forma incubator showed poor quality and other four embryos had good quality.

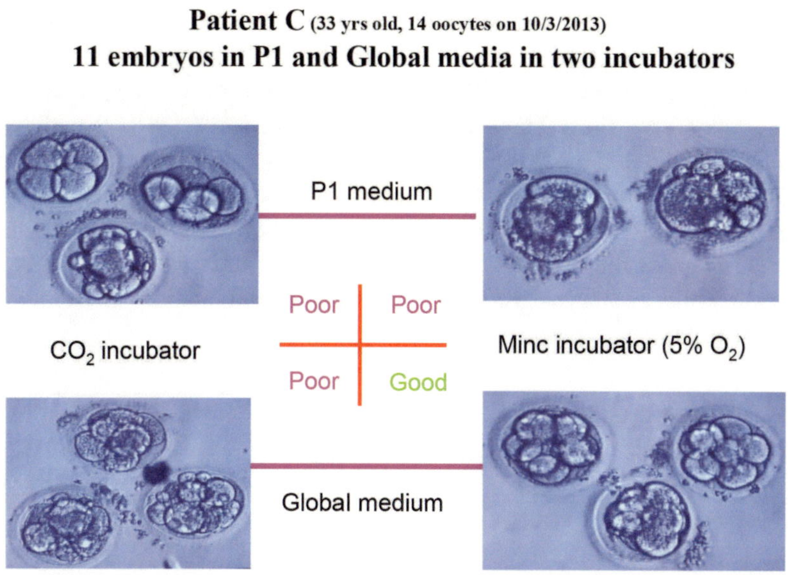

Figure 8. The eight embryos of a 33-year-old woman showed very poor growing with P1 medium in two incubators and global medium in big-box incubator. However, three good-quality embryos were obtained in the global medium with Minc incubator.

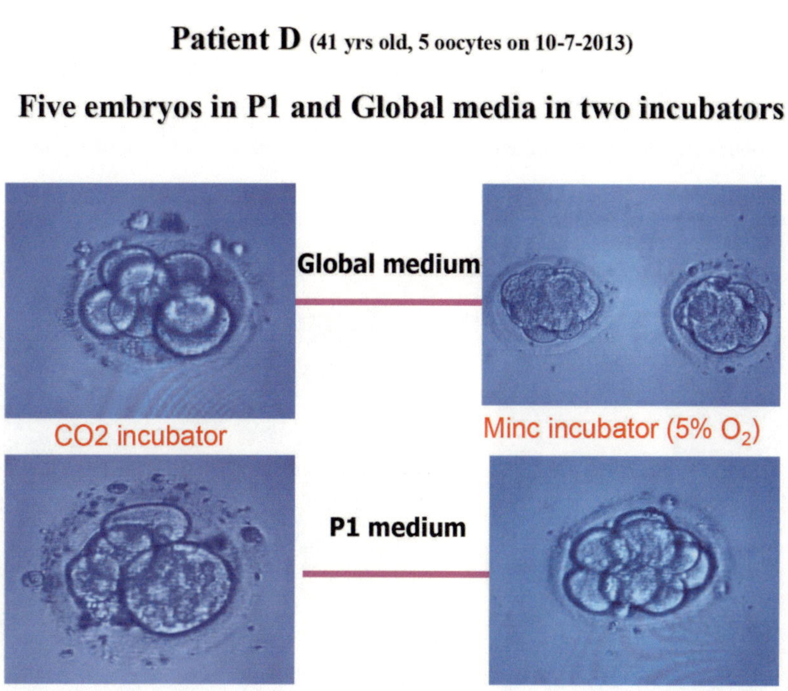

Figure 9. The four embryos of a 41-year-old woman showed very good growing with global medium in two incubators and Pl medium in the Cook Minc incubator. Only one embryo was of poor quality in the P1 medium with big-box incubator.

These results showed that the different patient's embryos had different responses to media. In order to compare large number of data, 1875 embryos of 174 patients were divided into four groups. The first group contains 45% (78/174) patient's embryos growing very well in either global medium or P1 medium. The second group contains 22% (38/174) patient's embryos growing well only in global medium with poor quality in P1 medium. The third group contains 21% (37/174) growing well in the P1 medium but poorly in the global medium and the fourth group contains 12% (21/174) not good growing in both P1 and global media (**Table 2**). In order to clearly show the data of table, a bar graph was drawn (**Figure 10**). We may very clearly see some patient embryos growing very well in global medium or P1 medium, which showed patient embryo selectivity.

Embryo quality in medium	**Patients/total patients (%)**	**Global medium**		**P1 medium**	
		Embryo number	**Top quality mean ±SD**	**Embryo number**	**Top quality mean ±SD**
Good in global and P1	78/174 (45%)	391/448	87.6 ± 16.3^{a}	359/425	84.5 ± 16.2^{a}
Good in global but poor in P1	38/174 (22%)	153/190	80.7 ± 22.8^{a}	67/205	32.8 ± 19.1^{b}
Good in P1 but poor in global	37/174 (21%)	51/185	27.7 ± 20.6^{a}	137/200	68.3 ± 22.5^{b}
Poor in global and P1	21/174 (12%)	30/105	28.8 ± 17.7^{a}	26/120	21.9 ± 20.9^{a}

Note: The same superscript in each row indicates no significant difference (P>0.05), and different superscript in each row indicates significant difference (P<0.05).

Table 2. Patient sibling embryos in response to different culture media.

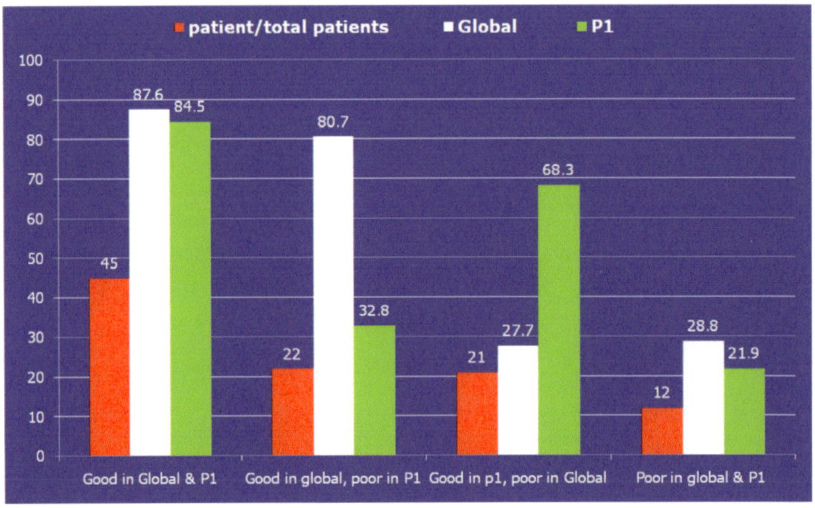

Figure 10. Growing distribution of patients' embryos in two media for culture. The first bar in each group represents percentage of patient's embryos in each group. P1 indicates P1 medium and G indicates global medium. The data indicate percentage.

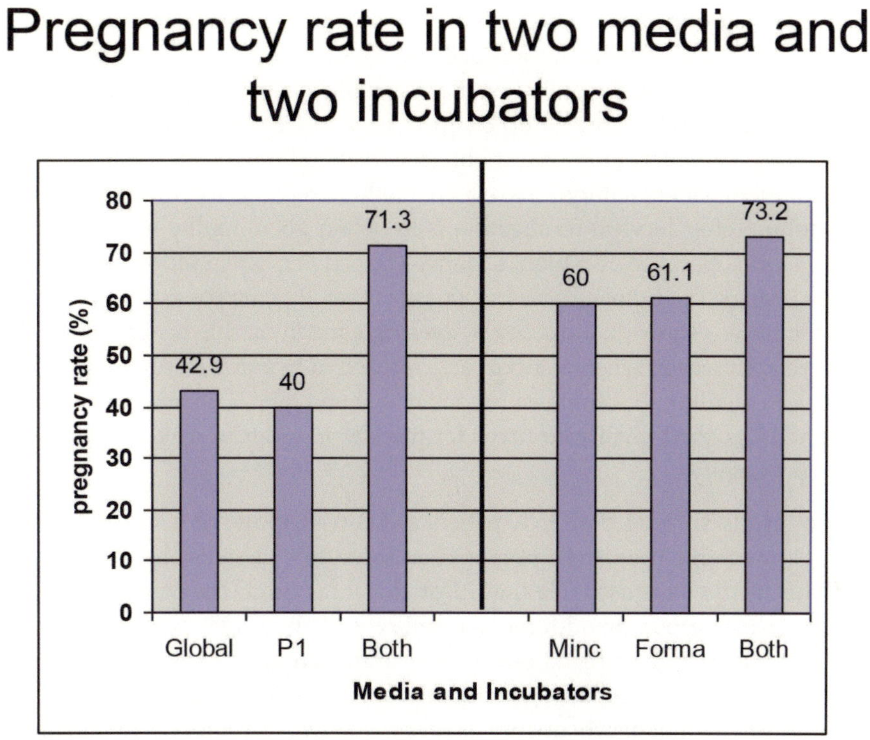

Figure 11. The statistics of patient pregnant rates in two media and two incubators.

The statistics of the pregnant rate showed 40% (10/25) in P1 medium and 42.5% (9/21) in global medium (P>0.05). However, when two media were used simultaneously for patient embryo culture, the pregnant rate significantly increased to 70.1% (122/174). At the same time, when two media were cultured in two incubators, it had a significant higher pregnant rate than in single incubator (73.2% vs. 60%, P<0.05, **Figure 11**).

5. Discussion

In the last near four decades, assisted reproductive technologies have been widely applied to the treatment for infertile couples to realize their dream to have baby in their family. However, the current successful rate is still kept in low level about 40%. Thus, vast efforts have been undertaken to improve IVF pregnancy rate by continuously improving and modifying in vitro culture medium system and innovating in embryo selection techniques such as time-lapse, preimplantation embryo diagnosis and screening (PGD/PGS). So far, numerous studies have been reported on different culture medium formulations and their effects on embryo cleavage and blastocyst formation [12]. Although current commercial culture medium composition varies widely, all of them may support human embryo in vitro culture growing very well. Thus, the selection of embryo culture medium depends on laboratory embryologist's favor and custom.

However, we are reporting a new observation which showed patient's embryo-specific differences in response to culture media in clinical IVF-ET. Our results indicated that some patient's embryos favored to grow in the global medium, while some patient's embryos preferred to live in the P1 medium and some embryos grow very well in both the global medium and P1 medium; some patient's embryos did not grow well in both P1 and global media, which means that different patient embryos have a favorable selectivity to culture medium. The aim of embryo culture after in vitro fertilization is to obtain good-quality embryos for transfer into women uterus. Because of patient's embryo selectivity, when all embryos of a patient are placed in a single medium culture, it is possible that all embryos are either very good or very poor. If embryos show poor quality in the single medium, this patient may be a failure in this IVF cycle. However, when embryos are cultured in two media, some embryos may be poor quality in a medium, but some embryo may be good quality in another medium. Thus, this patient still has good-quality embryos for transfer in order to make sure an increase in pregnancy opportunity.

Our statistic results showed that 45% patient's embryos grow very well in either global medium or P1 medium. Thus, the embryos from these 45% patients always grow very well no matter what media were used in either P1 or global medium. They are also easy to obtain successful pregnancy group. In addition, the embryos of about 12% patients could not grow well in both P1 and global media. These patients of this group are very difficult to get pregnancy because they cannot get any good-quality embryos for transfer using any medium. This may be due to patient oocyte quality or sperm quality. The embryos of remaining about 43% patients displayed a real medium selection. That means that 22% patient's embryos were growing very well only in P1 medium but poor quality in global medium, while the embryos of 21% patients grew well in the global medium but poorly in the P1 medium. Thus, we may obtain high-quality embryos from this 43% patient group by the selection of two culture media. In this way, the best estimation of IVF successful rate may reach to 45 + 43 = 88% of patients under the current IVF technology. In our statistics based on various ages of transfer embryo women, the pregnant rate of each group in two media and two types of incubators are listed in **Table 3**. However, this very high pregnancy rate resulted in 20.7% twin and 3.74% triplet baby birth, which showed that two medium cultures really increased transfer embryo implantation opportunity. In clinical practice, the number of transfer embryos should be reduced significantly accordingly.

Patient age	Transfer embryo no. and range	Pregnant no. and rate (%)
<28	1.98 (1–2)	20/23 (86.96%)
28–34	2.64 (1–3)	50/67 (74.63%)
35–27	2.94 (2–4)	24/33 (72.72%)
38–40	3.12(1–4)	21/32 (65.63%)
>40	3.81 (2–4)	9/21 (42.86%)

Table 3. The result of pregnancy with two media and two types of incubators for embryo culture and mixed embryo transfer.

Transferring embryos from two media may significantly improve human IVF pregnancy rate. Wirleitner et al. [17] ever reported an interesting observation in which the transfer of two embryos where one embryo was cultured in either medium resulted in a significantly high rate of twin pregnancies. Our research showed that two medium cultures might obtain 71% pregnancy rate. However, if single medium was used for culture, it may just produce about may produce about 40% pregnant rates. Using two media in one incubator for culture may increase to 60% pregnancy rate. When two media plus two incubators were used, the pregnancy might increase to 73%. Thus, the application of two media and two types of incubators may significantly improve human IVF/ICSI clinical pregnancy.

6. Conclusions

Patient-specific variability in response to commercially available media appears to play a significant role in clinic IVF practice, and the application of two media and two types of incubators for each patient embryo culture enables to ensure every patient to have sufficient high-quality embryos for transfer. The favorable response of individual patient's embryos to media and incubators suggests that in IVF clinic practice, using two media and two incubators for embryo culture could significantly improve IVF/ICSI pregnant rates.

Author details

Bin Wu[1*], Jinzhou Qin[2], Suzhen Lu[1], Linda Wu[1] and Timothy J. Gelety[1]

*Address all correspondence to: bwu13@yahoo.com

1 Arizona Center for Reproductive Endocrinology and Infertility, Tucson, Arizona, United States

2 Reproduction Medical Center, Luohu Hospital Affiliated to Shenzhen University, Shenzhen, Guangdong, China

References

[1] Brachetm A. Recherches sur la de"terminisme he're'ditaire de l'oeuf des mammife'res. De'veloppement in vitro de jeunes ve'sicules blastodermiques de lapin. Archives de Biologie (lie'ge). 1913;**28**:423-426

[2] Biggers JD. IVF and embryo transfer: Historical origin and development. Fertility Magazine. 2013;**16**:5-15

[3] Whitten WK. Culture of tubal mouse ova. Nature. 1956;**177**(4498):96

[4] Quinn P, Kerin JF, Warnes GM. Improved pregnancy rate in human in vitro fertilization with the use of a medium based on the composition of human tubal fluid. Fertility and Sterility. 1985;**44**(4):493-498

[5] Biggers JD. Thoughts on embryo culture conditions. Fertility Magazine. 2014;**16**:34-43

[6] Biggers JD. History of KSOM, a single medium for embryo culture. Fertility World. 2005;**3**:4-7

[7] Rieger D. A single medium can support development of human embryos to the blastocyst stage. Fertility World. 2005;**3**:24-27

[8] Edwards RG. Test-tube babies, 1981. Nature. 1981;**293**:253-256

[9] Gardner DK, Lane M. Embryo culture systems. In: Trounsoon AO, Gardner DK, editors. Handbook of In Vitro Fertilization. 2nd ed. CRC Press LLC; The United State of America 2000. pp. 205-264

[10] Fong C-Y, Bongso A. Comparison of human blastulation rates and total cell number in sequential culture media with and without co-culture. Human Reproduction. 1998;**14**:774-781

[11] Morbeck DE, Baumann NA, Oglesbee D. Composition of single-step media used for human embryo culture. Fertility and Sterility. 2017;**107**(4):1055-1060. DOI: 10.1016/j.fertnstert.2017.01.007

[12] Morbeck DE, Krisher RL, Herrick JR, Baumann NA, Matern D, Moyer T. Composition of commercial media used for human embryo culture. Fertility and Sterility. 2014;**102**(3): 759-766

[13] Aoki VW, Wilcox AL, Peterson CM, Parker-Jones K, Hatasaka HH, Huang I, Carrell DT. Comparison of four media types during 3-day human IVF embryo culture. Reproductive BioMedicine Online. 2005;**10**(5):600-606. DOI: 10.1016/S1472-6483(10)61667-7

[14] Chronopoulou E, Harper JC. IVF culture media: Past, present and future. Human Reproduction Update. 2015;**21**(1):39-55. DOI: https://doi.org/10.1093/humupd/dmu040

[15] Mantikou E, Youssef MAFM, van Wely M, van der Veen F, Al-Inany HG, Repping S, Mastenbroek S. Embryo culture media and IVF/ICSI success rates: A systematic review. Human Reproduction Update. 2013;**19**(3):210-220

[16] Swain JE. Optimal human embryo culture. Seminars in Reproductive Medicine. 2015; **33**(2):103-117. DOI: 10.1055/s-0035-1546423

[17] Wirleitner B, Vanderzwalmen P, Stecher A, Zech MH, Zintz M, Zech NH. Individual demands of human embryos on IVF culture medium: Influence on blastocyst development and pregnancy outcome. Reproductive BioMedicine Online. 2010;**21**:776-782